COLOURING

A Salon Handbook

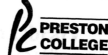

COLOURING
A Salon Handbook

Second Edition

Lesley Hatton

Longman

Longman
Longman Group Limited
Longman House, Burnt Mill, Harlow
Essex CM20 2JE, England
and Associated Companies throughout the world

Trademarks
Throughout this book trademarked names are used. Rather
than put a trademark symbol in every occurrence of a trademarked
name, we state that we are using the names only in editorial
fashion and to the benefit of the trademark owner with no intention
of infringement of the trademark.

First edition published 1986 by Collins Professional and Technical Books
Reprinted 1987, 1989, 1990, 1992 by BSP Professional Books
Second edition published 1995 by Longman

British Library Cataloguing in Publication Data
A catalogue entry for this title is available from the British Library.

ISBN 0–582–28759–6

Library of Congress Cataloging–in–Publication Data
A catalog entry for this title is available from the Library of Congress.

Typeset in 10/13pt Souvenir

Produced by Longman Singapore Publishers (Pte) Ltd.
Printed in Singapore

Contents

About This Book

This book is designed for every hairdresser working with hair colour. The information is written in a down-to-earth way which is easy to understand and provides answers to the questions you will ask. There are numerous diagrams to illustrate particular colouring techniques and summative at a glance charts which condense the important facts.

You will find this book essential reading if you are new to hairdressing or if you already have a sound knowledge of hairdressing but want to become a better colourist. The book provides the level of knowledge required for those involved in the training and education of hairdressers at foundation, intermediate and advanced levels.

There are short revision questions at the end of each chapter for you to test how much you have learnt (all the answers are in the text!) plus a selection of more challenging questions (requiring essay type responses) for the more advanced colourist. The glossary at the back of the book will serve as a quick reference guide to those words which may be new to you or to terminology you may have forgotten.

Colouring hair is a very interesting and rewarding part of a hairdresser's work. The best colourists have a sound theoretical knowledge which underpins their practical skills – this book will help you to become one of these people.

Acknowledgements

The following people kindly offered their valued opinions and help in the writing of this book:

Pamela Goff and The L'Oréal Technical Centre (London);
Clairol;
Wella (GB) Ltd;
Dr I.B. Sneddon and Dr R.E. Church gave permission to reproduce a photograph from their book *Practical Dermatology* (3rd Edition), published by Edward Arnold.

Lesley Hatton

Basic Facts

1.1 Hair facts

What is hair?

If you are to work successfully as a hair colourist, it is important that you fully understand the fibre with which you are working. Hair is a highly complex fibre and has a fascinating structure.

Hair is composed of a type of protein, called *keratin*, which is different from other proteins because it contains sulphur. The chemical composition of hair is shown in Figure 1.1. There are *three* different types of hair found on the human body:

- *Lanugo* hair is found on the human fetus before birth;
- *Vellus* hair is the fine downy hair found all over our bodies except the soles of our feet, palms of our hands and lips. (Yes, there are even hairs on our eyelids!);
- *Terminal* hair is the type that we deal with as hairdressers. It is coarser than vellus hair and is found on the scalp, on men's faces, under the arms and in the pubic region.

Hair can be classified into the following *ethnic* types and colouring can be carried out on all of them:

- Afro-Caribbean/Negroid
- Chinese/Mongolian
- European/Caucasian.

You will already be aware that hair also differs in texture and density. We use certain words to describe these differences in the appearance and feel of hair. We describe the texture of hair as curly, straight, thick, fine, coarse, etc., and the density of hair (i.e. how many hairs there are on the scalp) as thick, thin, fine, dense, sparse, etc. A natural redhead has about 90 000 hairs, while natural blondes have about 140 000 and brunettes fall somewhere in between. Therefore, natural blondes appear to have a greater

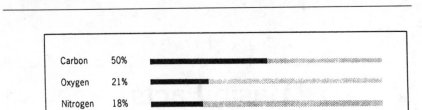

Carbon	50%	
Oxygen	21%	
Nitrogen	18%	
Hydrogen	7%	
Sulphur	4%	

Fig. 1.1 Chemical composition of hair.

density of hair but also tend to have the finest (smallest in diameter) hair. Incidentally, female hair is usually finer than male hair.

We also use words to describe the condition of a client's hair. Such words include dry, porous, sensitized, damaged, brittle, resistant, etc. We shall be looking at how hairdressers reach these conclusions in Chapter 2.

As the fibre we are dealing with is dead, there is nothing we can do to change how it grows. Cutting hair won't make it grow faster or thicker. Once hair has been damaged, it cannot be permanently repaired. The only way to change the quality of new hair is through diet and good hair-care routines.

How does a hair grow?

All hairs grow from a minute pit in the skin's surface called a hair *follicle*. The number of hair follicles we have is determined genetically and does not alter throughout our lives. However, whether a hair grows out from the follicle, and the type of hair produced, will change. For example, the vellus hair on a young boy's face alters as he reaches maturity to become terminal hair. Later on in life, the terminal hair on his scalp may be replaced by vellus hairs (male pattern baldness). The hair we see emerging from the scalp is dead but at the base of the follicle the hair is alive and actively growing.

There is a lot of activity at the base of the follicle and this area is called the *papilla*. It is here that cells are dividing and sub-dividing to produce hair as we recognize it. As the cells are going through this dividing process (called *mitosis*) they push the older cells upwards towards the opening at the scalp surface. It is also at the papilla that the hair's colour and shape is determined. Cells called *melanocytes* produce the natural pigment which determines the hair's colour. When these melanocytes stop producing the pigment, the hair from that particular follicle will emerge white, or technically speaking, colourless. The medical term for white hair is *canities*. The blood supply at the base of the follicle is extremely important as it is the blood which supplies the hair with everything it needs to grow, i.e. glucose, amino acids and oxygen. Lack of any of these nutrients due to, for example, the slimming disease anorexia nervosa, will result in hair of poor quality which may eventually drop out. Hormones, which are also transported around our bodies in the blood, affect hair growth too. Hormones cause hair to change from the vellus to the terminal type and vice versa and it is not uncommon for women to experience slight hair loss following childbirth as a result of the sudden change in their hormonal balance.

On average, hair grows approximately 1.25 cm (about half an inch) per month. This varies with the time of year (fastest in summer, slowest in winter). Therefore, clients having a permanent colorant application will need their regrowth re-touched after four to six weeks when the appearance of their natural hair colour at the roots will start to become noticeable.

On average, we lose about sixty hairs a day. These are shed naturally when we comb, brush or shampoo our hair. The reason we lose some hairs, but not all in one go (unless something is very wrong) is because we have a hair growth cycle. About 85% of the hairs on your head are actively growing and these hairs are described as being in the *anagen* stage of the growth cycle. The anagen stage can last up to seven years although it usually lasts two to three years. Once the hair has stopped growing it will reach the *catagen* stage. This is when the hair is dying and comes away from the base of the follicle and therefore its source of growth. About 1% of the hairs on our heads are in the catagen stage which lasts about two weeks. The follicle then rests for about three or four months and this is called the *telogen* stage. About 14% of our hairs are in this resting stage at any time. Following this rest, a new hair starts to grow and anagen starts again. This is shown in Figure 1.2.

To remember the hair growth cycle stages, use the word ACT to help commit it to memory.

Hair growth cycle stages:

A = Anagen
C = Catagen
T = Telogen

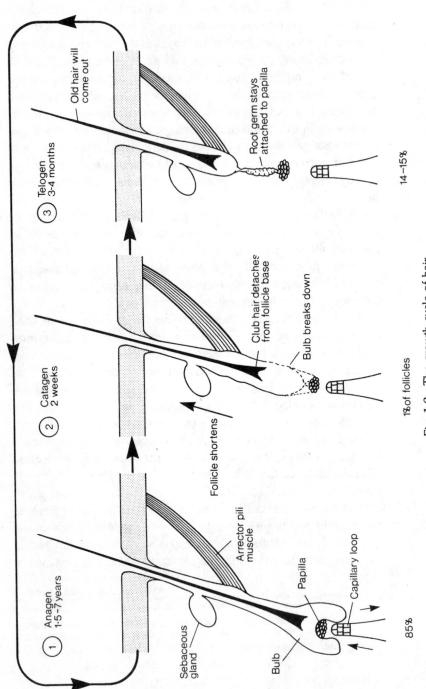

Fig. 1.2 The growth cycle of hair.

What is the structure of a hair like?

Hair is made up of three layers and can be likened to a pencil. The outside of the hair (the paint on a pencil) is called the *cuticle* and provides protection for the layers below. The next layer makes up the bulk of the hair (the wood of the pencil) and is called the *cortex*. The centre layer (the lead of the pencil) is called the *medulla*.

Figure 1.3 shows a hair which has been magnified over one thousand times. It would be impossible to see this detail with the naked eye. The scales you can see are one of several layers of the *cuticle*. European hair has about seven layers of these scales. Chinese hair has as many as eleven layers while Afro-Caribbean hair has fewer layers. The cuticle is completely colourless and the scales overlap with each other rather like the scales on a fish. The cuticle when it is lying flat and smooth, is responsible for making the hair shine as it reflects light. When the cuticle becomes damaged and worn, the scales become open and rough, and the hair will appear dull. A cuticle in this damaged state is referred to as being *porous* and this can affect hair colouring procedures and possible colour results: colorants on porous hair can fade quickly or 'grab' (colour is absorbed more quickly than expected). As the cuticle scales are transluscent, which means they allow light to pass through them, the colour we see is in the layer below the cuticle.

The layer below the cuticle, the *cortex*, makes up the bulk of a hair. The cortex is responsible for giving a hair its strength and elasticity and contains the natural colour pigment. The cortical fibres are rather like a bunch of straws held together by complex

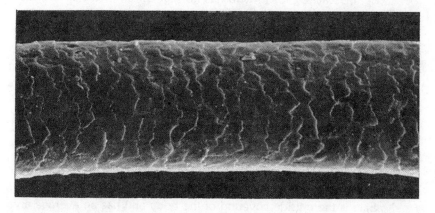

Fig. 1.3 A highly magnified hair (×1100).

bonds. The cortex is where all the chemical processes responsible for bleaching, tinting, perming and relaxing take place. Hair in good condition can stretch up to a third of its own length and then return to its original length. If the cortex becomes damaged, the hair will be weak, lifeless, lack bounce and may make some forms of colouring, such as bleaching, a very unwise course of action.

The natural pigment found in the cortex is deposited by the melanocytes. Melanocytes produce two types of pigment called *melanin* and *pheomelanin*. All natural hair colours are a combination of these two pigments. The differing amounts of these pigments result in the variations of natural hair colour we see about us. Melanin is the black and brown pigment while pheomelanin is the red and yellow pigment. Therefore, a person with dark hair will have mostly melanin whereas a person with fair hair will have mostly pheomelanin. Melanin is described as being *granular*. The word granular means the melanin molecules are like granules in appearance; large and easy for bleaches penetrating the cortex to find. Conversely, pheomelanin is described as *diffuse* because the molecules are small and scattered making them harder for the bleach to find. This is why dark hair lightens very quickly until it reaches the orange/yellow stage. When the melanocytes fail to produce the pigments, the hair will become colourless and will be seen as white. Because this process takes place at the base of the follicle, while the hair is forming, it is impossible for a person to go white overnight. In addition, there is no such thing as grey hair. We may think we see grey hair but it is simply an illusion created by seeing a combination of naturally coloured and white hair mixed together. If you don't believe this, try pulling out a single grey hair from someone's head and you'll discover that it is white! By the way, a person who has no pigment in their hair or skin is called an albino.

The centre of the hair is the *medulla*. The medulla serves no useful purpose to the hairdresser. It is basically an air space, which may, or may not, be continuous throughout the length of a hair. In fine hair, the medulla may be non-existent while in other hairs there may be two!

1.2 Skin facts

What is the skin?

Skin is the outside covering of the body and has an average area of over $1.6\,m^2$ ($18\,ft^2$) and an average weight of about $1.3\,kg$ ($6\,lb$).

Skin is attached to the underlying muscles by a layer of sub-cutaneous fat and consists of two main layers called the *epidermis* (outer layer) and the *dermis* (inner layer).

Figure 1.4 shows a generalized vertical section of the skin. This diagram includes all the relevant skin structures, although some would not be found on particular parts of the body (e.g. no hair follicles would be present if this diagram was showing the skin structure of the palms of the hands).

The skin is a protective layer with numerous nerve endings which tell us about our surroundings. If we feel too hot or too cold it is the blood vessels in the skin which help us reach normal body temperature again by dilating if the body is too hot and constricting if the body is too cold. The skin stores food in the form of fat, and can manufacture vitamin D (needed for healthy bones) and melanin (which gives us our natural skin colour and helps to protect skin cells from the sun's ultra-violet rays).

The epidermis

The *epidermis* is made up of five different layers. It contains no blood vessels and varies in thickness over our bodies from being as fine as a cigarette paper on our eyelids (0.1 mm thick) to the much thicker epidermis we have on the soles of our feet (about 2 mm thick). A superficial scratch or graze of the skin's surface will not bleed as long as the dermis has not been damaged because the epidermis contains no blood vessels. This is why chiropodists are able to safely cut away and remove hard skin from our feet without drawing blood.

The *five* layers of the epidermis are as follows:

Germinating layer (or basal layer)
The germinating layer is the bottom layer of the epidermis and is arranged as an orderly row of cells which is constantly dividing to form new cells. As new cells are produced, the old ones are pushed upwards to the surface of the skin to replace those which have been worn away. Small cells called *melanocytes* are found amongst the cells of this layer. Melanocytes produce the natural pigment of our skin and help protect our skin from the damage caused by the sun's rays.

Prickle cell layer
This layer is so-called because some of the soft nucleated cells have tiny outgrowths which give the cells a spiky appearance. It is

thought that melanin granules enter the cells through these outgrowths.

Granular layer
In this next layer the nuclei in the cells are breaking down and forming keratin, which causes the cells to die.

Clear or lucid layer
Above the granular layer is a harder, flattened layer of cells which contain keratin and have no nuclei or melanin granules. This gives rise to their clear appearance.

Horny or cornified layer
This is the outermost layer of the epidermis composed of flat, dead, scale-like cells which are constantly being rubbed off the body by friction from our clothes and off the scalp through the brushing of our hair.

The dermis

The *dermis* (or 'true skin') is between 1 and 4 mm thick and is made up of tougher more elastic tissue than the epidermis, containing numerous blood vessels and nerves. It is the different types of nerve endings in the dermis which carry messages to our brains and make the skin sensitive to pain, heat, cold and pressure.

You can see from Fig. 1.4 that the *follicle* is a downward growth of the germinating layer of the epidermis into the dermis. The hair grows from the epidermal cells at the base of the follicle surrounding the papilla. Attached to the side of the follicle is a *sebaceous gland* which produces and secretes an oily liquid called *sebum*. The sebum is secreted directly into the hair follicle and lubricates our skin and hair. Sebum also helps to waterproof our skin. Too much sebum makes hair greasy while too little causes the skin and hair to be dry. *Eccrine sweat glands* are found all over the body and secrete sweat which consists of 98% water and 2% sodium chloride (common salt). Eccrine sweat glands are coiled tubes leading to an opening (sweat pore) in the skin's surface. Sweating cools our bodies as the perspiration evaporates. Sweat glands are under the control of our nervous system. This is why we not only perspire when we are hot but also when we are nervous. *Apocrine sweat glands* are found in the underarm region and secrete directly into the hair follicle. The perspiration secreted from these special sweat glands is readily attacked by bacteria, which break it down, causing body odour. Hair follicles also have *arrector*

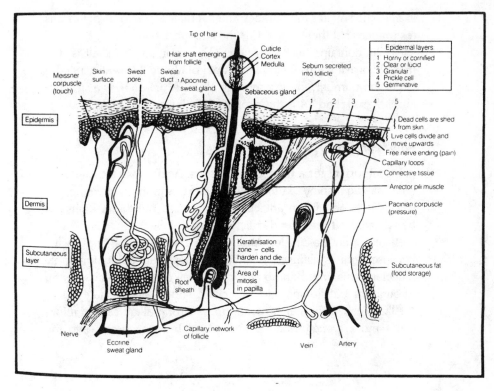

Fig. 1.4 A generalized vertical section of the skin.

pili muscles attached which contract when we are cold or frightened to cause the hair to stand erect and the skin to rise in a 'goose-pimple'. The standing up of the hair is an attempt to trap an insulating layer of warm air around the body but this is now quite ineffective because the evolution of human beings means that we are no longer hairy enough for this to work very well.

1.3 All about pH

What is pH?

The term 'pH' is simply a way of indicating how acid or alkaline something is. pH is expressed on a scale from 0 to 14, with 7.0 in the middle being the neutral point, where something is neither acid nor alkaline.

Acids contain hydrogen ions. The stronger an acid is, the greater the concentration of hydrogen ions it contains. A pH of below 7.0

is acid, the smaller the number, the stronger the acid. A pH of 2 is a stronger acid than 3, and 0 is the strongest acid.

Alkalis contains hydroxide ions. The stronger an alkali is, the more hydroxide ions it contains. A pH of above 7.0 is alkaline; the larger the number, the stronger the alkali. A pH of 10 is a stronger alkali than 8, and 14 is the strongest alkali (see Fig. 1.5).

Why is pH important to hairdressing?

pH is important for a number of reasons. Acids close the cuticle of hair, making it shiny. As the natural colour is in the cortex, the hair will look its best when artificial colour is also put there. Light will be reflected off the closed cuticle (see Fig. 1.5).

Alkalis open the cuticle, although this makes the hair appear dull because light is diffused (scattered rather than being uniformly reflected). It is important to allow the small colour molecules entry through the cuticle and into the cortex, and alkalis facilitate this.

Alkalis cause the hair to swell up. A strong alkali can therefore cause more damage than a strong acid because it gets into the

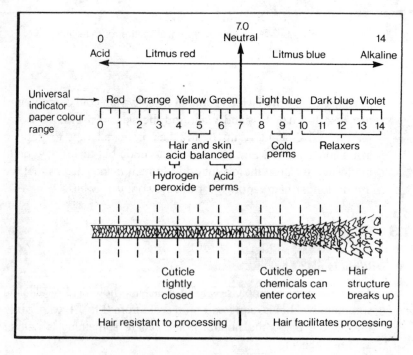

Fig. 1.5 Effect of pH on hair.

cortex easily (whereas the acid closes the cuticle and so cannot enter the cortex very quickly). Figure 1.5 shows how the hair swells and eventually breaks up.

To counteract damage to the hair when we use alkaline chemicals, we often use acid or anti-oxidant rinses. These close the cuticle and neutralize any remaining alkaline chemicals in the hair.

Acid-balanced products have the same pH as the hair and skin – with a pH of 4.5 to 5.5, average 5.4 – and so do not upset the natural pH.

1.4 Colour facts

We all take colour for granted. We look at things and know that they have a certain shade of colour – but what is colour?

Our natural daylight is referred to as 'white light', but it is itself a mixture of seven colours – red, orange, yellow, green, blue, indigo and violet. We see these seven colours, in this order, in a rainbow. To remember the order of the seven colours, remember the phrase '*Richard Of York Gave Battle In Vain*' – the first letter of each word being the first letter of a colour.

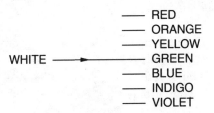

Fig. 1.6 Colour spectrum.

If something appears *white*, it is because all seven of these colours are being reflected to your eyes off the object that you are observing. If, however, an object appears as one of the seven colours, it is because that colour is being reflected to your eyes, while the other six colours are being absorbed (actually, a little of the colour on either side of the colour you see is also reflected). So, if you see orange, it is because orange is reflected to your eyes (with a little red and yellow) while the other colours are absorbed.

On the other hand, if something appears *black*, it is because all seven colours are being absorbed, so no colour is reflected to your eyes.

Colouring of hair

Hair colouring is achieved by the application of a pigment, or mixture of pigments, to the hair. Thus, unless bleaching is occurring at the same time (bleaching is the removal of colour), colouring involves the addition of colour to the natural pigments of the hair.

What is a primary colour?

This is a colour that cannot be produced by mixing other colours. In physics these colours are red, green and violet. In hairdressing, however, we are talking of pigments rather than pure coloured light. To a hairdresser the primary colours are *red, yellow* and *blue*. This is because we cannot make pigments of these three colours by mixing other pigments.

What is a secondary colour?

These are the colours that can be obtained by mixing primary colours together. Most of us mixed paints as children, and it is by mixing dyes together that the manufacturers develop their ranges of various shades.

Mixture of primary colours		gives secondary colour
Red + yellow	⟶	orange
Blue + red	⟶	violet
Yellow + blue	⟶	green

What is a complementary colour?

These are colours which are directly opposite each other in the colour circle (see Fig. 8.2 later in Chapter 8). They are also known as contrasting colours, and are important to colouring because they can mask unwanted colour. From the mixing of primary colours above, you can see that putting a blue rinse on hair with a lot of yellow in it can produce unwanted green! Unless it is St Patrick's day your client will not want this so, to overcome it, apply a red toner. The red is opposite to green in the triangle. Similarly, blue would remove unwanted orange.

Other information on colour

- Black is *not* a colour, but is a total absence of colour.

- White is a mixture of all the spectral colours – red, orange, yellow, green, blue, indigo, violet.
- Hues are full-strength spectrum colours (red, green, etc.).
- Tints are hues lightened by adding white.
- Shades are hues darkened by adding black.
- Pastels are hues which have been mixed with white and black.
- Tone is the intensity of the colour we see.

Salon lighting

The best source of light for hair colouring purposes is natural daylight so if it is available, please use it. When a natural source of daylight is unavailable or insufficient we need to resort to using artificial lighting. Lighting in a salon should provide sufficient illumination to allow people to work free from eyestrain (which can be caused by inadequate light or glare) and closely resemble natural daylight. If you intend colouring hair in artificial light it is important that you understand how it could cause you to misjudge what you are seeing. Have you ever bought clothes which seemed to be a different colour in the shop?

The two types of artificial lighting available are *tungsten filament bulbs* and *fluorescent tubes.* Tungsten filament bulbs are available in a range of colours, shapes and sizes. Some are made with plain, clear glass, others are coated (or frosted) to reduce glare or have special reflective surfaces for spotlighting displays. Filament bulbs have an average life expectancy of about 1000 hours but their efficiency deteriorates with age. They tend to give a reddish-yellow light with less blue and green than daylight so can be described as giving a 'warm' light. This makes hair colouring difficult because red shades of hair will appear redder ('warmer') under filament bulbs and ash/blue hair colours appear darker (and 'cooler') than in natural daylight. This means that a client could see the new hair colour very differently under tungsten filament lights as compared to its appearance in natural daylight.

Fluorescent tubes are much more efficient than filament bulbs and will last up to five times longer. They are cheaper to run because a greater amount of the electrical energy is converted into light energy and not wasted as heat, but they are more expensive to buy and install. They give a diffused light which is free from glare and they cast little shadow. Diffusers can be fitted to provide 'softer' light and reduce the chance of glare if viewed from directly below. The colour of the light produced by fluorescent tubes varies according to the type of fluorescent powder used to coat the inside of the tube and can be a bluish white to a warm white which is very similar to daylight. 'White' fluorescent tubes have less red and yellow than daylight making blues and greens look brighter and reds shades duller and darker. A *warm white* fluorescent tube is the best type of fluorescent tube and far better for hair colouring than a filament bulb because it is so similar to daylight.

Hair colours are often described as being 'warm' or 'cool'. Colours categorized under the headings of 'cool' and 'warm' are shown in Fig. 1.7.

Tips for working with colour

- Do not have too many colours in the salon as they can upset your judgement of hair colour.
- Competing colours can leave an after-image in the eyes so salon walls should be a pastel colour, ideally with a matt finish.
- If you have tinted lenses in your glasses remember to remove them when matching colours or invest in a pair which have a graduated tint that is clear glass at the bottom.
- If you are matching colours, rely on your first impression because the longer you look at closely matching colours, the more they tend to blend together.

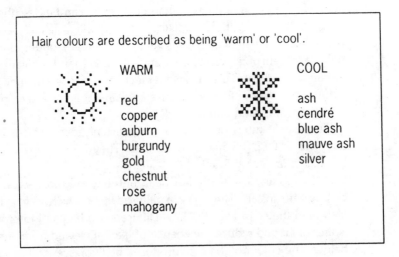

Fig. 1.7 Warm and cool colours.

1.5   Revision questions

1   What is the name of the protein from which hair is made?
2   What are the three types of hair found on the human body?
3   What are the ethnic classifications for hair?
4   What is the name of the pit in the skin's surface from which a hair grows?
5   Where would you find the hair papilla?
6   What is the name of the process by which the cells divide to produce a hair?
7   What do melanocytes produce?
8   What is the medical term for white hair?
9   Approximately, how much does a hair grow in a month?
10   On average, how many hairs do we lose naturally a day?
11   What are the three stages of the hair growth cycle called?
12   Name the three layers of the hair.
13   What is the outermost layer of the hair called?
14   In which layer of the hair do chemical processes take place?
15   In which layer of the hair will the natural colour pigment be found?
16   Name the two colour pigments found in the hair.
17   Name the pigment which is described as granular.
18   Name the pigment which is described as diffuse.
19   Name the two layers of the skin.
20   How many layers make up the uppermost layer of the skin?
21   What is the name of the natural oil produced by the sebaceous gland?
22   Which type of sweat gland is found all over the body?
23   What is the name of the sweat gland found in the underarms?
24   What is the best source of light for hair colouring?
25   If artificial light has to be used when colouring hair, which type is recommended?

1.6   Advanced questions

1   Describe the structure and growth of hair with the aid of diagrams.
2   Describe the skin structure and draw a diagram showing a hair and its appendages.
3   Describe the effect that alkalis and acids have on hair and state the pH of the skin, hair and hairdressing products.
4   Describe the different sources of artificial lighting available and their effects when working with hair colour.

Precautionary Tests and Safe Working Guidelines

You are responsible for the safety and well-being of your client. Many of the chemicals used in salons are potentially hazardous, so it is important to minimize risks by taking the necessary precautions and carrying out appropriate tests.

It is important to remember that clients are not always aware of the products they have on their hair, or of the significance of answering your questions truthfully. We have all come across the client who has a regrowth and insists that her hair is natural and has never been tinted! Unfortunately, not all products used previously on the hair are as obvious to detect as this . . .

2.1 Porosity test

What is it?

The porosity test checks for external damage, i.e. the degree of damage to the cuticle.

What does 'porosity' mean?

The porosity of the hair determines the cuticle's ability to allow the absorption and passage of moisture and products. Hair porosity varies from person to person, but it increases when the cuticle becomes damaged and open.

As shown in Fig. 2.1(a), in non-porous hair the cuticle scales lie flat against the hair shaft. Because the scales are flat they reflect light evenly, making the hair appear shiny. Such hair is less likely to be damaged when brushed or combed, because the cuticle scales will not be 'caught' as easily.

In porous hair, the cuticle scales are open and protruding from the hair shaft, as shown in Fig. 2.1(b). Because they form an

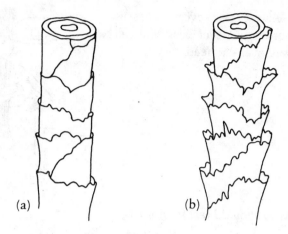

Fig. 2.1   (a) Non-porous and (b) porous hair.

uneven surface to the hair, light is diffused rather than reflected, making the hair appear dull. Porous hair will allow products to enter quickly, resulting in more rapid chemical processing. If the porosity is uneven along the hair shaft it may result in uneven colouring.

What makes hair become porous?

Damage to the cuticle can be caused in two ways:

(1) Chemically – by using alkaline products which open the cuticle, leaving the hair susceptible to further damage, both external and internal;
(2) Physically – by the over-use of heat (heated rollers, tongs, holding the dryer too close to the hair, sun, etc.). General physical abuse such as harsh brushing and back-combing will also open the cuticle, leading to cuticle abrasion.

Remember that the oldest hair will be most damaged, i.e. the points.

How do I test for porosity?

Take a few strands of hair and hold firmly near the points. Slide your fingers down the hair shaft to the roots. The rougher it feels, the more porous the hair.

Always test several areas as porosity is never even and will vary over the head.

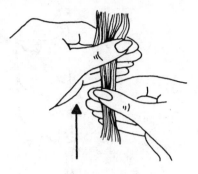

Fig. 2.2   Porosity test.

Why should I test for porosity?

An increase in porosity will mean that products may behave differently than expected. Colour molecules will enter the hair shaft very easily and may become more deeply lodged than anticipated. This means that temporary and semi-permanent colours could stay in the hair longer than usual. This is often referred to as colour 'grabbing'. Because the degree of porosity varies along the hair shaft, the colour could also be uneven and patchy.

However, it can also have the opposite effect by allowing colour molecules to escape more readily. This means that tints will fade very quickly, especially red shades.

Can the porosity of the hair be improved?

Yes, but only temporarily. Conditioners help smooth the cuticle, coating the hair with a film of wax or oil, helping to 'fill in' the places where the cuticle scales have actually broken away. Remember that some conditioners could create an unwanted barrier on the hair, preventing other products from working effectively when colouring.

2.2   Elasticity test

What is it?

The elasticity test is a way of assessing the degree of internal hair damage, i.e. to the cortex.

What does 'elasticity' mean?

Elasticity is the ability of hair to be stretched and then return to its original length. A hair in good condition can stretch up to one third of its own length and then return to its original length. Hair is more elastic when wet. Poor elasticity is always accompanied by a damaged, porous cuticle.

What makes hair lose its elasticity?

Poor elasticity is due to the cortex being damaged. It is mostly caused by chemical processes such as perms, tints and bleaches, but occasionally by severe physical abuse.

How do I test the elasticity of hair?

Take a strand of hair and hold firmly at each end with the thumb and forefinger. Pull gently between the fingers and see how much the hair stretches and springs back. It takes experience to be able to judge this accurately.

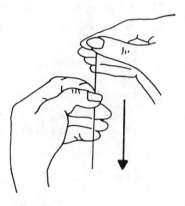

Fig. 2.3 Elasticity test.

Just like an old elastic band, damaged hair will snap when stretched.

Why should I test for elasticity?

Because, besides causing further unwanted damage, you may end up with uneven colour results which will fade quicky and appear 'flat' (matt).

Can internal hair damage be repaired?

No. The damage is irreversible because the chemical bonds in the cortex have been broken. However, products are available which reform the damaged bonds temporarily and are sometimes applied before colouring to help the hair withstand further treatment.

2.3 Skin test

What is it?

A skin test indicates whether or not the client is allergic to the para-compounds contained in oxidation tints. The word para refers to the main active ingredient of most tints, which are either para-phenylenediamine (black shades) or para-toluenediamine (brown shades). It is the para-phenylenediamine which has the greatest tendency to produce an allergic reaction in people. Because of this its use in hair colours has been banned in Germany, France and Austria (although companies from these countries still produce it for our use!). It has been shown to induce cancer in laboratory tests on animals, but the quantity required to do so is unlikely to be encountered by the client or hairdresser. (See Fig. 2.4 for an example of an allergic reaction to a tint.)

The skin test is also known as the patch test, sensitivity test, predisposition test or Sabourand-Rousseau test.

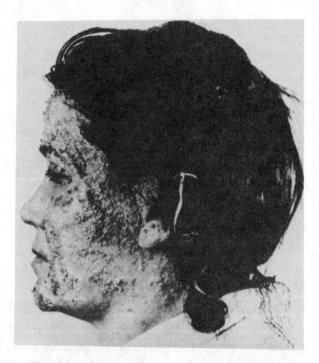

Fig. 2.4 Hair dye dermatitis. An example of a bad allergic reaction to a tint. Prevent this from happening in the salon by giving a skin test. (From *Practical Dermatology* by I.B. Sneddon and R.E. Church (3rd Edition). Publisher: Edward Arnold).

What do I need to carry out a skin test?

peroxide (20 vol/6%)
tint
bowl and brush
gown and towel
record card
measure
collodion (optional)
spirit (surgical, eau de cologne)
cotton wool

How do I carry out a skin test?

- First protect client with gown and towel.
- Mix a small amount of tint (i.e. 2 cm or 1 capful) with equal parts of peroxide.
- Cleanse either the inside of the elbow or behind the ear using cotton wool and spirit. Pat dry.
- Place a smear of the tint (about the size of a penny) on the cleansed area and allow this to dry naturally *or* cover with collodion. (When possible, use the shade intended for the client's hair, otherwise use the darkest shade as it contains more para-compound).
- Record relevant information on card (e.g. date, client's name and address, product used).
- Tell the client to leave the test area undisturbed for at least 24 hours. However, if the client should experience any discomfort, swelling, itching, etc. he or she should remove the tint and apply a soothing lotion such as calamine. If there is no reaction, it can be presumed safe to proceed with the tint application.

A positive reaction (redness, swelling, irritation) indicates that the client is sensitive to the product and under *no* circumstances should a tint application take place. About one in *every* twenty-five people is allergic!

If the reaction is positive, clients may have the following instead:

highlights, lowlights, vegetable colours, bleach, temporary colours, some semi-permanents.
(N.B. Check product formula of semi-permanents as some contain small amounts of para-compounds.)

Because product formulae change and client sensitivity is unpredictable, manufacturers advise that a skin test is done *every* time a client wishes to have a tint.

In the most severe allergic reactions, besides a skin irritation, there may be difficulty in breathing. Without medical attention the person could even die. The type of people most likely to get such a reaction would be those who suffer from asthma or hayfever. If they should experience difficulty in breathing ask them if they have any anti-histamine tablets, which would relieve the symptoms. An ambulance should be called if the client has a bad reaction. Do not rely on the condition correcting itself.

Legally, *you* are responsible for the safety of the client.

2.4   Incompatibility test (1.20 test)

What is it?

This test indicates whether or not any products previously used on the hair will react unfavourably with the products you intend to use. It is specifically used for testing for the presence of metallic salts contained in some colouring preparations, such as colour restorers and compound henna. Any colouring system which uses hydrogen peroxide, such as bleaches and oxidation tints, will react violently, damaging both the hair and scalp.

What do I need to do an incompatibility test?

glass container
20 vol/6% peroxide
*ammonium hydroxide (0.880)
hair samples
sellotape
record card

*If ammonium hydroxide is not available in the salon, perm lotion may be used instead.

What do I do?

- Prepare the hair samples by cutting from an unnoticeable area and secure at root end with tape. You may need more than one sample.
- Mix together twenty parts of peroxide with one part of ammonium hydroxide.

- Immerse sample(s) into solution. Leave for 30 minutes.
- Check the sample for the presence of bubbles, and feel the container to see if it is warm. The sample may also change colour. Any sign of effervescence, heat, etc. indicates that it is a positive reaction. This would mean that the hair has metallic salts on it, making it unsafe to use any product which is mixed with peroxide (i.e. tint, bleach).

The reason for adding ammonium hydroxide is that it speeds up the reaction; peroxide alone would be too slow.

2.5   Test cutting/colour test

What is it?

The test cutting is a way of assessing colour results before the application of the intended product to the entire hair. A test cutting can be carried out to test the results of temporary, semi-permanent and permanent colours.

What do I need to do a test cutting?

the product(s) to be used
bowl and brush
graduated glass measure
hair samples
sellotape
record chart

What do I do?

- Prepare hair samples by cutting hair from unnoticeable areas and secure at root end. You may need several.
- Mix product(s) and immerse samples into labelled bowls.
- Process, rinse and record results.

A test cutting clearly indicates to you and the client exactly how the hair will respond to the colours used. Damaged hair has uneven porosity and will result in an uneven colour. A test cutting will help you decide whether the hair should be subjected to further colour treatment and what will give you the best results.

2.6   Strand test

A strand test is performed to monitor colour development and results. To check colour results on a regrowth application, the colorant is cleaned from the hair using the back of a comb or a piece of damp cotton wool. For full head colour applications, the colorant is wiped from a small mesh of hair using damp cotton wool so that the colour of the roots can be compared to that of the lengths and ends. The area selected for the strand test is usually the crown but there will be occasions when other parts of the head will be more appropriate for checking colour results.

2.7   Safe working guidelines (including COSHH)

The Control of Substances Hazardous to Health (COSHH) regulations introduce a new legal framework for controlling people's exposure to hazardous substances through their work activities. Some types of hair colouring agents are classified as *irritants* so it is very important to follow manufacturers' instructions to ensure the safety and well-being of your clients and those working alongside you.

- Remove chunky jewellery, bulky sweaters, etc. and protect the client with gown and towels – you are liable to pay for any damage.
- *Always* read and follow manufacturers' instructions, they are designed to work and be used in a specific way – formulations may change without your having noticed.
- Ensure that you and the client have both agreed on the final colour result *before* starting.
- Measure accurately – don't guess.
- Carry out appropriate tests – don't take risks.
- Keep record cards up to date – don't imagine that you will remember.
- Wear rubber gloves when colouring – your hands are your livelihood.
- Products can irritate – avoid inhaling fumes.
- If a product accidentally enters the eye, immediately flood with water. Seek medical advice if irritation continues.
- Accidental stains on the skin should be removed as soon as possible, using a product designed for this purpose.

2.8   Recording client information

Why should records be kept?

It is essential that a record is kept of any colouring that a client has had. There are a number of reasons:

- You will not remember what products were used, or how and when you used them;
- When you next see the client you can check on the product performance;
- You will know when the client last had a skin test;
- If you are away, there will be no guess-work involved for the colleague attending to your client;
- The clients will be aware that they are being treated professionally.

What information should be recorded?

Client's name	Include surname, forename (or initials) and their title (i.e. Mr, Mrs, Ms, Miss, Dr, etc.)
Address	You will be able to check the address with your client to ensure you have the correct card.
Date of appointment	This enables you to see when the client visited the salon for colouring or skin tests.
Stylist	This tells the salon who the client's stylist is.
Scalp	The scalp condition should be recorded, e.g. sensitive, dry and scaly, oily, psoriasis, etc.
Condition/quality of hair	Gives details of hair, e.g. resistant, porous, damaged, etc.
Colouring technique	Records highlights, regrowth application, touch-colour, bleach and toner, etc.
Products	Sets out quantities, strengths and types of products used.
Development	Shows whether an accelerator was used, how long the product was on the hair, etc.

Result   Perhaps the result was too pale or too
                              ash. This should be recorded so that
                              changes can be made next time.
*Special information   Conversation topics, client's interests,
                              etc.

*You can increase the quality of service and business by making a
note of personal details of each client. These might include notes
such as the client drinks white coffee with one sugar, will need an
ashtray, likes to be called by his/her forename, etc. This will give
clients a feeling of belonging to your salon, and they will marvel at
your amazing memory!

How can this information be recorded and stored?

Information can be recorded in two ways:

(1) Writing the information on a record card (see Fig. 2.5);
(2) Entering data into a microcomputer.

Record cards are generally stored in a filing box or cabinet.
Salons file the cards in alphabetical order of the client's surnames,
so they can be retrieved easily and quickly. Cards should be refiled
after use.

Although a computer can store a great deal of information about
the salon and its clients, it may not be practical for keeping this
type of information. The stylists in a salon would have to know
how to call up the information, and unless you have a powerful

NAME						SPECIAL INFORMATION	
ADDRESS							
DAYTIME TELEPHONE NO.							
DATE	STYLIST	SCALP	HAIR	TECHNIQUE	PRODUCTS	DEVELOPMENT	RESULT

Fig. 2.5   Client record card.

machine, this may also take several valuable minutes to do. However, there may be rapid advances in technology, so try to visualize the micro working in a salon.

When should colouring information be recorded?

Colouring information should be recorded immediately after the colouring appointment. Don't leave it to the end of the day because you may forget what was used. Skin tests should also be recorded, with confirmation that the test was either positive or negative.

2.9 Revision questions

1 What would be the appearance of the cuticle if the hair was described as porous?
2 What can make hair become porous?
3 What is the purpose of carrying out an elasticity test?
4 What can make hair lose its elasticity?
5 What is the purpose of carrying out a skin test?
6 How frequently should a skin test be performed?
7 What are the indicators of a positive reaction to a skin test?
8 What is the purpose of performing an incompatibility test?
9 What would you expect to see if an incompatibility test proved to be positive?
10 What is the purpose of carrying out a test cutting?
11 What is the purpose of carrying out a strand test?
12 What do the initials COSHH stand for?

2.10 Advanced questions

1 Explain the importance of performing precautionary hairdressing tests in relation to COSHH and manufacturers' instructions.
2 Describe how you would perform a skin test and state the advice you would give the client.
3 Explain the importance of maintaining client information records for colouring and describe a record system with which you are familiar.
4 Describe the tests you would perform to determine the condition of a client's hair before proceeding with a colouring service and how your findings could influence:

(a) your chosen application technique
(b) the type of product used
(c) the final result.

3

Types and Performance of Hair Colorants

Colouring products vary in their formulae and in their application. Some require preparatory mixing and skilled application, while others are ready to use and easy to apply. In this part of the book, these differences will be explained and because the indiscriminate use of certain colorants may have dermatological or toxicological side-effects, the ingredients and characteristics are included.

The complicated terminology used by scientists, manufacturers and indeed some hairdressers to describe various colouring products can be bewildering. It is often difficult to perceive the differences between for example, a 'colour shampoo', 'colour restorer', 'cosmetic colorant' or 'rinse'. Much of this confusion can be attributed to manufacturers and hairdressers alike, who promote a particular colouring service or product using words which appeal to current trends. For example, some hairdressers promote semi-permanent colorants as 'vegetable colours' because this conjures up an image of a 'healthy' or 'back to earth' product which is free from synthetic ingredients.

Hairdressers often use a special vocabulary for promoting hair colour to clients and replace some words used for describing colouring techniques and products with more attractive terms. Examples of this practice are the common use of the terms 'pre-lighten' instead of bleach, 'tint' instead of dye and 'direct colour' instead of semi-permanent.

3.1 Temporary colorants

Temporary colours very simply cause an *instant change* in hair colour. They are designed to be brushed or rinsed off the hair and at most, last until the hair is next shampooed. Temporary colours are ideal for introducing colour to colour-shy clients and are extremely useful for creating stunning fashion looks and interesting effects for hairdressing competition work. They work most effectively on lighter shades of hair but are equally popular with hairdressers for producing rich tones on darker hair. One manufacturer promoted its range of temporary colours by the slogan 'a rinse brings it, and a rinse takes it away' which aptly describes how temporary colours work. However, if temporary colours are applied to very porous hair, the result may not rinse off the next time the hair is shampooed. This is because the large molecules of this type of colorant adhere to the cuticle scales of the hair as shown in Fig. 3.1. If the cuticle scales are open (porous), these molecules will remained trapped for longer because they are able to enter further into the layer than if the cuticle was closed.

Temporary colorants are used to:

- Beautify hair colours and enhance a slightly dull shade;
- Restore the natural hair colour after exposure to sunlight;
- Eliminate yellow in white hair;
- Restore colour between semi-permanent or permanent tint applications;
- Correct 'off-shades' produced by other colouring techniques and products;
- Give hair a new tone – 'just to see what it looks like'.

The formulae characteristics of temporary colours are that they:

- Are easy to eliminate by shampooing the hair;

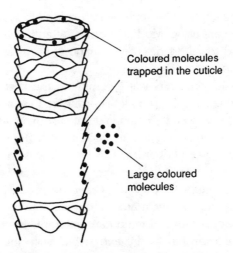

Coloured molecules trapped in the cuticle

Large coloured molecules

Large colour molecules adhere to the cuticle. Applied in final coloured form. Chemically, they are azo-dyes. Last until the hair is next shampooed but could last longer on porous hair.

Fig. 3.1   Effect of temporary colour on hair.

- Have sufficient resistance to friction (to avoid loss on clothes, hats, pillowcases, etc.);
- Are sufficiently colour-fast in rain or in contact with perspiration.

The formulation of temporary colorants (by the expert chemists employed by hairdressing product manufacturers) often creates difficulties because the product may need to have a dual purpose. For example, coloured setting lotions and mousses need to consist of a combination of dyestuffs and film-forming anionic polymers, to provide the 'hold' expected from such a styling product. The predominant dyestuffs of temporary hair colorants include azo and azine derivatives, methyl violet, methylene blue, indoamines and indophenals.

There are many different types of temporary colorants which fall in and out of popularity as fashion and social trends change.

Types of temporary colorants include:

- Coloured setting lotions, gels and mousses containing plasticisers
- Coloured hair sprays
- Coloured powders or liquids which are diluted with water
- Shampoos containing temporary dyes
- 'Paints' and crayons.

The application of temporary colorants will depend upon the type you are using. Most are applied after the hair has been shampooed and towel-dried. (Towel-drying is necessary to avoid diluting the colour effect.)

Manufacturers will recommend the best method of application but usually the product is distributed evenly through the hair with the hands and a comb. You may sometimes find it useful to apply coloured setting lotions by emptying the product into a tint bowl and using a tint brush. This technique is recommended if you want to concentrate the application on particular areas of the hair (such as a regrowth) or when using the product to correct 'off-shades' where only certain areas require colouring.

Some types of temporary colorants are designed to be applied when the hair is dry and styled as in the case of coloured hair sprays, 'paints' and crayons. Sometimes, as in the case of coloured hair sprays, it is possible to remove by brushing, temporary colours applied to dry hair. Over-use of temporary colorants can result in colour build-up which dulls the hair.

Summary of temporary colorants:

- Convenient and easy to use;
- No commitment required from client;
- Most effective on lighter shades of hair;
- Ineffective for complete coverage of white hair;
- Easily rinsed out of the hair;
- Large colour molecules coat hair shaft;
- May have dulling effect if over-used;
- Cannot lighten hair;
- Can 'grab' on porous hair and last longer than required;
- Instant result – no development time necessary.

3.2 Semi-permanent colorants

Semi-permanent colorants are designed to cause a change in hair colour which resists *four to six shampoos* and are capable of darkening and changing the tone of hair. They are ready to use, require no mixing and are easy to apply. Semi-permanent colorants are sometimes called 'direct colours' because technically speaking they are not mixed with an oxidant (i.e. hydrogen peroxide) in order to develop the colour.

They are usually applied to freshly shampooed hair which has been towel-dried (to prevent dilution of the product) and require rinsing from the hair after the recommended development time has elapsed (which can vary between 10–30 minutes). Semi-permanents are applied to the hair either using a tint brush, sponge, applicator bottle or directly from the tube or bottle. Some hairdressers apply these to the hair while the client is positioned at the backwash basin, while others prefer to have their client sitting upright in a styling position.

Semi-permanent colorants work by depositing colour molecules in the hair which penetrate the cortex (as shown in Fig. 3.2) where they combine with the hydrogen bonds. These colour molecules need to be comparatively small to be able to penetrate the cuticle and enter the cortex and the product has a pH of between 8 to 9 to aid this penetration. Each time the hair is shampooed, some of the colour molecules are replaced by water causing the colour to weaken. By the fifth or sixth time the hair is shampooed, the colour should be completely lost. Small molecules may be able to enter the hair shaft easily but are lost relatively quickly.

On unevenly porous hair, the resultant colour effect may be patchy and uneven and last longer than expected. This is because

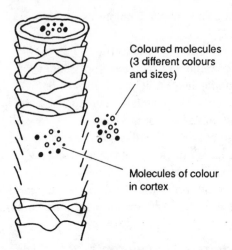

Coloured molecules
(3 different colours
and sizes)

Molecules of colour
in cortex

Mixture of different sized and coloured molecules penetrate the
cortex because they are applied in an alkaline form (which opens
the cuticle). Chemically, they are nitro-dyes. The colour fades each
time the hair is shampooed but should last between four and six
shampoos.

Fig. 3.2   Effect of semi-permanent colour on hair.

the colour molecules will penetrate further into the hair structure
and certain ingredients found in semi-permanents react selectively
on different portions of a damaged hair. For example, the red
colour molecules found in semi-permanents are the smallest so will
enter the hair structure easily. However, because they are small,
they are the first to be lost from the hair.

Semi-permanent colorants are used to:

- Add various tones to hair colour, i.e. gold, ash, copper, red,
  burgundy;
- Darken hair and effectively disguise up to 30% of white hair;
- Rid hair of unwanted tones, i.e. correcting yellow tones in white
  hair to achieve a more flattering pastel tone;
- Brighten and enhance hair colour between permanent tint
  applications.

The formulae characteristics of semi-permanent colours are that
they:

- Are unlikely to cause scalp irritation and allergy;
- Have sufficient resistance to friction, sunlight and shampooing;

- Are unlikely to affect the future chemical processing of hair, e.g. perming.

The predominant ingredients of semi-permanent colorants are nitro-phenylenediamines (which give red and yellow colours) and anthraquinones (which give blue colours). The different combinations of these ingredients in semi-permanent products result in a wide range of colours from which to choose.

Types of semi-permanent colorants include:

- Liquids and creams
- Non-drip foams and mousses
- Shampoos containing semi-permanent dyes.

The application of semi-permanents will mainly depend on the type of product you are using and whether the manufacturer has designed it to be applied directly to the hair from the product's container. Some hairdressers like to apply liquid form semi-permanents from a tint bowl using a tint brush, while others prefer to use a sponge or applicator bottle. Semi-permanents are often packaged to enable the hairdresser to apply the colorant from the container instead of transferring the contents to a tint bowl or applicator bottle. The product should not be applied directly to the skin or scalp because semi-permanent colorants can stain the skin. For this reason, protective gloves should always be worn by the hairdresser.

Summary of semi-permanent colorants:

- Convenient and easy to use;
- No commitment required from client;
- Coverage of white hair (up to 30%);
- Variation in porosity can lead to uneven or patchy results;
- Small colour molecules penetrate the cortex;
- No pre-mixing required (unless mixing one or more shades together);
- Development time between 10–30 minutes on average but less time needed for freshly permed or porous hair;
- No adverse effect on the condition of the hair;
- Gradual wash-out of colour (usually lasts four to six shampoos);
- Cannot lighten hair;
- Skin test may be required if it contains a para-dye.

3.3   Quasi-permanent or cosmetic colorants

Quasi-permanent or cosmetic colorants, as they are often called, have recently gained in popularity but were also available in the 1960s and 1970s. They are non-lightening colorants and can be described as a cross between semi-permanent and permanent colorants. This description is appropriate because they are mixtures of nitro-phenylenediamines and/or anthraquinones (found in semi-permanent colorants) and para-dyes (found in permanent oxidation tints) and require mixing with an oxidizing agent (hydrogen peroxide). The semi-permanent part of a cosmetic colorant will gradually wash out of the hair but the loss of colour will not be complete because of the permanence of the para-dyes. Consequently, these colorants will last longer (on average up to 12 shampoos) and will result in a regrowth.

The durability of the colour will depend greatly on the condition of the client's hair and the type of shampoo which is used, but an obvious regrowth will only be apparent if the colour applied is noticeably darker than the client's natural hair colour.

The strength of hydrogen peroxide added to cosmetic colorants is relatively low, typically a strength of between 1–3% (6 to 10 vol). Manufacturers may call the oxidant a 'colour developer', 'colour activator' or 'colour releaser' to emphasize the difference in strength of the oxidant compared to that used with permanent oxidation tints and to avoid using the words 'hydrogen peroxide', a solution which may be perceived as being damaging to the hair.

The addition of an oxidant 'locks' the colour in the cortex of the hair (see Fig. 3.3) but because the hydrogen peroxide is of such a low strength, it has little effect on the natural pigment in the hair. Colour results will gradually fade each time the hair is shampooed (like a semi-permanent colorant) but will also produce a regrowth. Cosmetic colorants should be treated in a similar manner to permanent oxidation colorants and a skin test is essential because some people are allergic to colorants containing para-dyes.

Cosmetic colorants are used to:

- Beautify and enhance natural hair colours and add shine;
- Refresh the colour of old highlights;
- Create natural translucent coverage for up to 50% of white hair;
- Restore natural hair colour and pre-colour (colour correction);
- Revive faded colours between permanent oxidation tint applications.

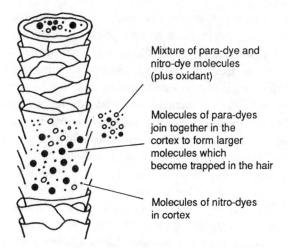

Mixture of para-dye and
nitro-dye molecules
(plus oxidant)

Molecules of para-dyes
join together in the
cortex to form larger
molecules which
become trapped in the hair

Molecules of nitro-dyes
in cortex

Mixture of different sized molecules enter the cortex and are
oxidized by hydrogen peroxide. Chemically, a mixture of nitro-dyes
and para-dyes. The nitro-dyes are gradually lost each time the hair
is shampooed. The para-dyes remain in the cortex resulting in
regrowth.

Fig. 3.3   Effect of quasi-permanent colour on hair.

The formulae characteristics of cosmetic colours are that they:

● Have sufficient durability and resist removal through several
shampoos.

The predominant ingredients of cosmetic colorants are mixtures of
nitro-phenylenediamines and/or anthraquinones and para-dyes.
Special conditioning agents may be included to add shine and
lustre to the hair. All cosmetic colorants require mixing with an
oxidizing agent which is a low strength hydrogen peroxide solution.

Types of cosmetic colorants include:

● Creams or liquids
● Liquids which become gel-like when mixed with the oxidant.

The application of cosmetic colorants will depend on the manufacturers' instructions and the type of hair to which you are applying
the product. When applying this type of colorant to freshly permed
hair you may be instructed to apply it quickly as a shampoo onto
damp hair, while untreated hair may require application to dry,
unwashed hair. For subsequent applications, manufacturers usually

recommend that the colorant is applied to the root area first, allowing development to take place for about ten minutes before taking it through to the lengths and ends of the hair.

When using this type of product to refresh the colour of old highlights, a shorter development time will be recommended than the average 15 minutes required for natural hair. If using this product to refresh already tinted hair which has faded, care should be taken in the selection of the colour to ensure it is a good match. To restore natural colour in lightened hair, natural and warm shades should be selected, and for use as a pre-colour (during colour correction) warm tones should be used.

The hair will need to be rinsed once the colour has developed and this is done by adding a little warm water to the hair at the backwash basin and massaging into a lather to loosen the colorant from the hair (this is called *emulsifying* a colour) before rinsing until the water runs clear.

Summary of cosmetic colorants:

- Careful application required if applying to regrowth area;
- Colour activated by hydrogen peroxide;
- Careful measurement and mixing of product required (usually 2 parts of oxidant to 1 part of colorant – a ratio of 2:1);
- Translucent coverage of up to 50% of white hair;
- Comprehensive colour range but cannot lighten hair;
- Grows out (regrowth will be more noticeable if colour used is much darker than client's own hair colour);
- Development time of between 5–20 minutes;
- Skin test required;
- Colour molecules completely penetrate the cortex.

3.4   Permanent oxidation colorants

Permanent oxidation colorants (or tints) are the only colorants capable of giving permanent hair colour, in an infinite variety of shades, with complete coverage of 100% of white hair. The availability of high quality, sophisticated products in comprehensive colour ranges has never been better. They are referred to as oxidation tints because they require the addition of hydrogen peroxide (an oxidizing agent) to bring about the chemical reaction which 'locks' the colour into the cortex of the hair.

An older term which is not often used these days to describe oxidation tints is 'para tints'. This description owes its origins to the fact that the first colorants of this type contained substances called *para*-phenylenediamines (black) and *para*-toluenediamines (brown). Since the manufacture of the first oxidation colorants, additional chemicals have been added to give a much wider range of colours and improve performance.

It must be remembered that oxidation tints contain chemicals which can cause dye dermatitis, so a skin test should be carried out before every tint application. A few people are allergic to this type of colorant and a sudden allergy could develop even though a client may have had the same tint applied for many years. Reasons for not using a permanent oxidation colorant are shown in Fig. 3.4.

Oxidation tints are mixed with hydrogen peroxide and it is the addition of this, in various strengths, which makes the dual action of dying and lightening possible. Tints are applied to unwashed, dry hair because the stimulation of the scalp and consequent removal of sebum caused by shampooing can cause irritation and discomfort for the client when the tint is applied. Many hairdressers prefer to comb the hair before a tint application rather than use a brush because the physical action of brushing can also make the scalp more sensitive to the chemicals. Oxidation tints need to be applied carefully, using a tint brush, to ensure that the colorant is only applied to the desired parts of the hair. A noticeable regrowth will appear within four to six weeks so subsequent 're-touching' of the roots is necessary to maintain the colour.

Permanent oxidation tints work by depositing small colourless molecules in the hair which penetrate the cortex. The pH of oxidation tints is about 9–10, and this level of alkalinity helps to open the cuticle and aids the penetration of the colorant. During

---

A permanent oxidation tint should **not** be applied if:

- no skin test has been carried out
- the skin test showed a positive reaction
- the scalp or hair show the presence of infection or infestation
- there are cuts and abrasions present on the scalp
- the hair condition is too poor to take a chemical service
- the selected target colour is unsuitable

Remember! If in doubt, don't apply a tint.

Fig. 3.4 Reasons for NOT tinting hair.

the development time, which is usually between 30–45 minutes, the colourless molecules coalesce (join together) to form large colour molecules which become trapped in the cortex because they are too large to be washed from the hair. This chemical reaction is called *polymerization* and is shown in Fig. 3.5.

Permanent tints are used to:

- Completely disguise white hair;
- Lighten hair;
- Darken hair;
- Change the tone of the hair;
- Produce a 'permanent' result (but a regrowth will appear after four to six weeks which will require periodic colouring).

The formulae characteristics of permanent tints are that they:

- Are capable of simultaneous bleaching and colouring;
- Are able to colour hair to all possible tones;
- Have sufficient durability so that one application lasts for between four and six weeks;

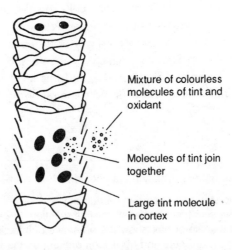

Mixture of colourless molecules of tint and oxidant

Molecules of tint join together

Large tint molecule in cortex

Small colourless molecules enter the cortex and are oxidized by hydrogen peroxide. The molecules coalesce (join together) to form large molecules of colour which are trapped in the hair. This chemical reaction is called polymerization. Chemically, they are para-dyes. Colour is permanent, resulting in a regrowth.

Fig. 3.5 Effect of permanent oxidation colour on hair.

- Cover white hair with a variety of shades, particularly natural shades.

The predominant ingredients of permanent oxidation tints include combinations of different chemicals including para-phenylene-diamines (black), pare-toluenediamines (brown), meta-dihy-droxybenzene (grey), para-aminolphenol (reddish-brown) and meta-phenylenediamines (brown). These chemicals are aromatic compounds belonging to three major chemical families: the diamines, the aminophenols (or amino naphtols) and the phenols (or naphthols).

Formulations of permanent oxidation colorants include:

- Liquids
- Creams
- Oil-based types (which 'gel' when mixed with the oxidant).

All permanent oxidation colorants need to be mixed with hydrogen peroxide. The strength of the hydrogen peroxide to be used with the tint will be stated in the manufacturers' instructions. The strength may vary between 3% (10 vol) and 12% (40 vol) depending on the product being used and the intended target colour. The use of higher strength hydrogen peroxide leads to greater lightening effects but should only be used if recommended by the manufacturer because the subtle tonal values of tints will be reduced or even completely lost if the strength of the hydrogen peroxide is too high.

Darker hair (i.e. brown) will be more difficult to lighten than hair which is lighter (dark blonde). It may only be possible to achieve up to two shades of lift on naturally dark hair when using a permanent oxidation tint. On lighter hair, it may be possible to achieve up to three shades of lift. There are special 'high-lift' tints available which are designed to achieve natural blonde shades and these are generally mixed with higher strength hydrogen peroxide than would normally be used. 'High-lift' tints will only achieve their maximum lift of 3–4 shades on hair which is no darker than dark blonde. If a client wishes to be a lighter shade than can be achieved with a tint, they will need their hair pre-lightened (with bleach) to remove the unwanted depth of colour and to prepare it for the application of a toner. Following the development and subsequent rinsing off of the bleach, a toner can be applied to the bleached hair, in the form of a permanent oxidation tint, to produce the desired colour tones. Attempts at using 'high-lift' tints on hair which is too dark, will result in colours which are too warm (i.e. too red or gold) and darker than desired.

Summary of permanent oxidation colorants:

- Careful application required;
- Colour activated by hydrogen peroxide;
- Careful measurement and mixing of product required;
- Coverage of up to 100% white hair;
- Comprehensive colour range; can lighten, darken and change tone;
- Grows out;
- Development time usually between 25–45 minutes;
- Skin test required;
- Colour molecules completely penetrate cortex;
- Can cause deterioration of the hair's condition.

3.5 Bleach

Bleaching is the removal of natural hair colour. The chemical reaction takes place in the cortex of the hair where the colour molecules (melanin and pheomelanin) are oxidized by the bleach to form a colourless molecule called *oxy-melanin* (Fig. 3.6).

Natural hair colours depend on the quantity of pigment and its distribution. The natural pigment of dark hair will consist mainly of melanin (black and brown) pigment. This type of granular pigment is easily oxidized and reacts favourably with bleach products, changing to oxy-melanin before the pheomelanin pigment is affected. Pheomelanin (red and yellow) pigment is more diffuse (smaller and scattered in the cortex) and will only be oxidized by the bleach when all the melanin has been changed to oxy-melanin.

It is this phenomenon which enables hairdressers to control the bleaching of hair. By purposely halting the bleaching process and thus the 'disappearance' of the diffuse pigment, various degrees of lightening can be achieved revealing tones from red to very pale yellow. These lightening degrees are known as bleach bases (or lightening tones) as expressed in Fig. 3.7. These lightening tones act as the 'undercoat' for the toner so it is important that the bleaching process is halted at the correct stage (see [4.10] – Bleach bases for toners). Failure to achieve the sufficient degree of lightening will result in unwanted tones 'showing through' the

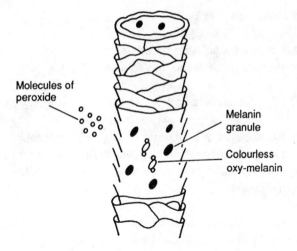

Molecules of peroxide

Melanin granule

Colourless oxy-melanin

Applied as an alkaline which aids penetration into the cortex. Natural pigment is oxidized to form colourless oxy-melanin. Melanin is removed first, followed by pheomelanin. Permanent colour resulting in a regrowth.

Fig. 3.6 Effect of bleach on hair.

	Bleach bases	Corresponding depths
Progressively lighter	reddish	5
	reddish/orange	5−6
	orange/red	5−6
	orange	6−7
	orange/yellow	7−8
	yellow/orange	7−8
	yellow	9
	pale yellow	10
	very pale yellow	10+

Fig. 3.7 Bleach bases and their depths.

toner. This can be imagined by using the example of trying to paint a door white which has been treated with a red undercoat. The resultant colour will be pink because the white paint will not cover the red undercoat paint sufficiently.

If the bleach is allowed to work on the hair for too long, resulting in the hair being too light, the toner applied will be too pale and will not 'hold' in the hair because too much pigment will have been removed.

Bleach is used to:

- Give hair a lighter appearance;
- Prepare the hair (by lightening) for the application of a toner.

The formulae characteristics of bleaches are that they:

- Are capable of lightening natural hair pigment;
- Have a consistency which aids their application;
- Can be sufficiently controlled to achieve different degrees of lightening.

There are many different forms of bleach available for professional use and all of them are oxidizing agents. Bleaches use the decomposition of hydrogen peroxide (supplied in either liquid, crystal or powder form) to supply the amount of oxygen needed to lighten hair. Hydrogen peroxide alone can be used to lighten hair (it was first introduced for this purpose by E. H. Thiellay, a London chemist and Léon Hugot, a Parisian hairdresser in 1867 at the International Exhibition in Paris) but this is a very slow process. If two shades of lift were required, a 20 volume hydrogen peroxide solution would have to be left on the hair for about 12 hours! Therefore, hydrogen peroxide needs to be mixed with an alkaline substance to speed the release of oxygen. A substance which speeds up a reaction but remains unchanged itself at the end of the reaction is called a catalyst.

Types of bleaches include:

- Powder or paste
- Emulsion
- Oil
- Lightening shampoos
- Lightening setting lotions.

Powder bleach

Powder bleach can lift hair by four to six shades and consists of *ammonium carbonate* and *magnesium carbonate*. When the powder is mixed with hydrogen peroxide it forms a smooth paste which is thin enough to be applied easily to the hair but thick enough not to run. The ammonium carbonate speeds the release of the oxygen and the magnesium carbonate helps to control the release of the oxygen. A swelling agent, such as carboxymethyl cellulose or a vegetable gum, is often added to bleaching powders to improve their consistency and slow down drying out and possible flaking once they have been applied. Small quantities of blue or violet colorants may also be added to help eliminate unwanted yellow tones in the resultant shade.

Some clients may experience a 'tightening' or 'burning' sensation of their scalp during the development of the bleach as it dries. For clients with sensitive scalps, an emulsion bleach should be considered.

Emulsion bleach

Emulsion bleaches have an oily appearance and when mixed with hydrogen peroxide form a gel which is easy to apply to the hair. Bleaching power is increased by the addition of powders known as 'activators' or 'boosters' and some emulsion bleaches can bleach hair up to six shades lighter.

These powders come in sachets and usually contain either *potassium persulphate* or *ammonium persulphate* which release enough additional oxygen to make the lightening process more effective. Conditioning agents, such as cetrimide, are usually present in emulsion bleaches to help reduce damage to the hair.

Emulsion bleach works as well as powder bleach but is more comfortable for the client because it does not dry out and tighten the scalp.

Oil bleach

Oil bleach is a soluble oil which is mixed with hydrogen peroxide, immediately before it is applied, to form a transparent or translucent gel which is easy to apply. Oil bleach is only capable of lifting the hair two or three shades and tends to induce yellow tones in the hair. Emulsion or powder bleaches should be used when greater lightening power is needed.

Lightening shampoos

A lightening shampoo (or bleach bath) is a mild form of bleach used when gentle lightening is required. It is made by mixing one part of shampoo, one part 6% (20 vol) hydrogen peroxide, one part water and one part of powder bleach. Lightening shampoos can be used to brighten naturally blonde hair but are more commonly used to 'clean out' unwanted colour build-up caused by temporary and semi-permanent colorants. Lightening shampoos can also be used for removing unwanted ash tones from bleached hair (see Chapter 8).

Lightening setting lotions

Lightening setting lotions contain plastic polymers and emollients normally found in setting lotions plus hydrogen peroxide, which is normally up to 3% (10 vol) in strength. These lotions are applied like normal setting lotions to shampooed, towel-dried hair and give progressive bleaching results when applied regularly (e.g. once a week).

The application of powder, emulsion and oil bleaches is always to dry, unwashed hair. Emulsion, powder and oil bleaches are most suited to being applied with a tint brush whereas bleach baths could be applied (to damp hair) using an applicator bottle or sponge.

Summary of bleaches:

- Careful application necessary;
- Pre-mixing required;
- Careful measurement and mixing of ingredients required;
- Some bleaches are capable of lifting colour up to six shades;
- Grows out (a regrowth will appear and require subsequent lightening);
- Lightening is observed during development – lightening process is halted when the bleach is rinsed from the hair;
- The high pH of bleach affects the condition of hair;
- No skin test is required unless an oxidation tint is to be applied as a toner after the bleach has been rinsed from the hair;
- Can irritate the scalp.

3.6 Vegetable colorants

Henna

The use of henna dates back thousands of years. It is known that the ancient Egyptians used it for colouring their hair, nails and palms of their hands. Henna is known as *khenna* to Egyptians, its Indian name is *mendee* and it is called *al khanna* in Arab countries.

Henna is a small shrub (*Lawsonia inermis*) with tapering branches and whitish bark and is cultivated in India, Tunisia, Arabia and Iran. The leaves of the *Lawsonia inermis* are dried and crushed to make a greenish-yellow powder which is then mixed with hot water to form a thick paste. Sometimes, additional ingredients such as acetic acid (to make the colour browner) are added to the mixture.

It is left on the hair for between 30 minutes and two hours and wrapping the hair with a plastic cap and towel helps to intensify the colouring effect. It is not uncommon for women in the Middle East to apply a henna paste to their hair which is left overnight. It will take two to three days before the final shade will be seen because henna is a progressive colorant which means it is slowly oxidized by the oxygen in the air.

When used on dark hair, henna produces various shades of 'orange-brown' but if it is applied to white hair an unattractive 'carrot' shade is produced.

The active ingredient in henna is *lawsone* but because henna also contains *tannin*, the hair is left with a certain degree of 'stiffness'. It is a totally natural product but its popularity fluctuates. The henna paste affects the hair by coating the cuticle and depositing colour in the cortex (Fig. 3.8) and should be treated as a permanent colorant because a regrowth will appear. As henna

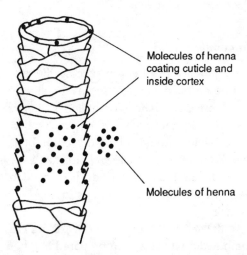

Molecules of henna coating cuticle and inside cortex

Molecules of henna

Henna coats the cuticle and enters the cortex. A natural colorant which is permanent and results in a regrowth. Can interfere with the penetration of chemicals such as permanent wave lotion.

Fig. 3.8 Effect of henna on hair.

coats the cuticle of the hair unevenly and penetrates the cortex, it tends to hinder the penetration of permanent wave lotions making successful perming difficult. It is the coating of the henna on the cuticle that gives a smooth surface to the hair, making it reflect light and shine.

Summary of henna:

- Preparation and application can be messy;
- Powder is mixed with hot water (and optional ingredients) to form a thick paste;
- Penetrates and coats the hair shaft;
- No skin test necessary – it is a natural product;
- Development time between 30 minutes and two hours (or even overnight);
- Helps to give hair shine;
- Grows out (a regrowth will appear);
- Unattractive shades produced on white hair;
- Progressive form of colorant – final shade not reached immediately;
- Cannot lighten the hair;
- Interferes with the penetration of other chemicals such as permanent wave lotions.

See compound henna [3.7].

Camomile

Camomile is a plant which successfully grows throughout Western Europe and is generally used as a culinary herb. However, it can also be used as a hair colorant and is often contained in proprietary shampoos for those who want to revive their naturally blonde hair.

The active ingredient of the colorant is yellow and is called *trihydroxyflavone*. To use camomile as a rinse, the dried camomile flower heads must be infused (like making tea) in boiling water. Once the mixture is cooled, it is strained and then poured through the hair.

To make a paste, the flower heads are crushed with kaolin into a fine powder which is then prepared like henna.

Summary of camomile:

- Can be applied as a rinse or as a paste;

- Dried flower heads infused by the addition of boiling water or crushed with kaolin into a fine powder before mixing with hot water;
- Molecules too large to enter the hair shaft;
- Camomile coats hair with a yellow cast;
- No skin test required;
- Must be done regularly to maintain colour;
- Does not cover white hair;
- Natural product.

3.7 Metallic colorants

The use of metallic or metallized dyes is as ancient as the use of henna. They have tended to disappear from the market except for the type called 'hair colour restorers' or 'progressive dyes' which are sold as colorants to be applied daily at home. They are not used by hairdressers as they are incompatible with all hairdressing processes which involve the use of hydrogen peroxide. These processes include oxidation tints, quasi-permanent colorants, bleaches and perms (hydrogen peroxide is the most commonly used oxidant found in neutralizer solutions).

Metallic dyes usually contain lead and silver salts but sometimes copper, nickel, cobalt and bismuth are added to vary the tones achieved. Lead salts are included in acetate or nitrate form. They are referred to as 'progressive' because the dye needs to be applied daily and slowly turns white hair a greyish colour before taking on a dark (but dull and flat) leaden colour after exposure to oxygen in the air. The metallic salts coat the cuticle and can penetrate the cortex. If the hair does come into contact with hydrogen peroxide, the metallic salts act as a catalyst, causing immediate breakdown of the oxidant and consequent damage to the hair (see [2.4]).

Compound henna is the natural henna powder combined with various metallic salts to produce a full range of colours which were very popular in salons throughout Western Europe in the early twentieth century. The application of compound henna also renders the hair unfit for future treatment with any product incorporating the use of hydrogen peroxide.

3.8 Types and performance of colorants at a glance

Fig. 3.9 will enable you to see at a glance the types of colorants available and their performance. Test yourself by covering

	Ingredients	Types available	How it works	Preparation
TEMPORARY	Rinses – methylene blue, methyl violet, acid, azo-dyes in setting lotions, lacquer, etc.	Gels, mousses, setting lotions, crayons, sprays, concentrated liquids, 'paints'	Large molecules coat hair shaft and are attracted to acid groups. Colour coats cuticle in plastic form.	No preparation unless in concentrated form.
SEMI-PERMANENT	Nitro-phenyl-enediamines (red-yellow). Anthraquinones (blue).	Liquid, cream and mousse	Three different sized molecules enter through cuticle to combine with hydrogen bonds in cortex. Water replaces the colour molecules with each shampoo.	No mixing required (unless two shades are to be mixed together).
QUASI-PERMANENT	Mixture of nitro-dyes and para-dyes.	Liquid, cream and oil-based ('gelling') formulae	Colour enters cortex where the para-dye molecules join together and are trapped. The nitro-dye molecules are replaced by water each time hair is shampooed.	Colorant is mixed with low strength hydrogen peroxide usually at a ratio of 1 part of colorant to 2 parts of oxidant – see manufacturers' instructions.
PERMANENT	Para-dyes (paraphenyl-enediamines/para-toluenediamines) or meta-dyes (metadihy-droxybenzene).	Liquid, cream and oil-based ('gelling') formulae	Small colourless molecules are oxidized in cortex to form coloured molecules which are trapped (polymerization).	Mixed with hydrogen peroxide according to manufacturers' instructions.

Fig. 3.9 Types and performance of colour – at a glance.

Application	How long it lasts	Advantages	Disadvantages
Either to dry or damp hair (depending on product). Can be used on all or part of the hair.	Until the hair is next shampooed.	No skin test required. Easy to apply. Instant result. Washes out with next shampoo.	Does not cover white hair. Can dull the hair. Will last longer than expected on porous hair.
Hair is shampooed and towel-dried. Applied directly from container or applicator bottle or with a tint brush or sponge.	Colour is gradually lost each time the hair is shampooed. Lasts for four to six shampoos – longer on porous hair.	Normally, no skin test required (but check manufacturers' instructions). Easy to apply. Can cover up to 30% white hair.	Can only disguise up to 30% white hair. Cannot lighten hair. Will last longer on porous hair. Development time necessary. Can stain skin and scalp.
Applied the same as a tint (for regrowth) or like a shampoo to damp hair. See manufacturers' instructions.	The nitro-dyes are lost each time the hair is shampooed (on average 12 shampoos) while the pare-dyes remain permanent.	Longer lasting results than semi-permanents. Covers up to 50% white hair. Easy to apply.	Skin test required. Regrowth will require subsequent colouring to sustain colour. Development time necessary. Can only disguise up to 50% white hair.
Applied to dry, unwashed hair with a tint brush. Careful application required.	Until it grows out. Results in a regrowth.	Can lighten, darken and change tone. Wide range of colours. Can cover 100% white hair.	Skin test required. Affects condition of hair. Time consuming. Regrowth will require subsequent colouring to sustain colour.

	Ingredients	Types available	How it works	Preparation
BLEACH	Oxidizing agent such as hydrogen peroxide or magnesium peroxide. Catalysts which speed release of oxygen.	Powder/paste, emulsion, oil, lightening setting lotion and shampoo	Bleach enters cortex and changes natural pigment to colourless compound (oxy-melanin).	Mixed to manufacturers' instructions'. Lightening setting lotion ready to use. Lightening shampoo is 1 part each of shampoo, oxidant, water and powder bleach.
HENNA	Ground leaves of the *Lawsonia inermis* shrub. Active ingredient is lawsonia.	Powder (Compound henna contains metallic dyes)	Penetrates hair shaft and is slowly oxidized by oxygen in the air (so is progressive). Coating on cuticle increases shine.	Powder mixed with hot water to form a paste. Additional ingredients may be added.
CAMOMILE	Dried flowers from camomile plant. Active ingredient is trihydroxyflavone.	Available as flower heads or in powder form (crushed flower heads mixed with kaolin)	Molecules coat cuticle with yellow cast. Hair must be treated regularly to sustain colour.	Dried flower heads infused with hot water or crushed with kaolin and mixed with hot water to form a paste.
METALLIC DYE	Metallic salts such as lead, silver, copper, etc.	Liquid. Not produced for professional use, e.g. Grecian 2000	The metallic dyes adhere to the cuticle giving it an unnatural and dull appearance.	Ready to apply. No mixing required.

Fig. 3.9 Continued

Application	How long it lasts	Advantages	Disadvantages
Applied to dry, unwashed hair with a tint brush. Careful application required.	Until it grows out. Results in a regrowth.	No skin test required. Can achieve up to six shades of colour lift.	Affects condition of hair. Time consuming. Regrowth will require subsequent colouring to sustain colour.
Applied to damp hair with a tint brush.	Gradually fades. Results in a regrowth.	No skin test required. Natural product. Makes hair shine.	Processing time lengthy. Difficult to rinse out of hair. Interferes with penetration of chemicals. Can leave hair 'stiff'.
Applied as a final rinse or as a paste which is then rinsed from the hair.	Fades. Requires subsequent applications to sustain colour.	No skin test required. Natural product.	Requires subsequent application to sustain colour. Not suitable for dark hair.
Applied daily to white hair and combed through. It is not rinsed out of the hair.	Until it grows out. Results in a regrowth.	No skin test required. Inexpensive. Easy and quick to apply.	Unattractive colour results. Hair unfit for future services involving the use of hydrogen peroxide.

some of the boxes to see how well you can remember the information.

3.9 Revision questions

1 State which layer of the hair the following types of colorants affect:

    (a) temporary
    (b) semi-permanent
    (c) quasi/cosmetic
    (d) permanent (oxidation) tint
    (e) bleach.

2 Name two vegetable colorants.
3 In which hair colouring process is oxy-melanin produced?
4 From which plant is henna obtained?
5 What is the active ingredient of camomile?
6 In which type of colorant would you find azo-dyes?
7 What is the expected lasting time of the following colorants:

    (a) temporary?
    (b) semi-permanent?
    (c) quasi/cosmetic colorant?

8 Which of the following types of colorants do not require a skin test to be carried out:

    (a) bleach?
    (b) temporary colour?
    (c) semi-permanent?
    (d) quasi/cosmetic colorant?
    (e) henna or camomile?

9 Which type of colorant is capable of successfully covering 100% white hair?
10 What type of colorant causes polymerization to occur?
11 What is compound henna?
12 What is the maximum amount of lift which can be achieved by a bleach?

3.10 Advanced questions

1 State the colouring services which could be safely recommended to a client who has shown a positive reaction to a skin test.

2 Describe (with the use of diagrams) how the following types of hair colorants affect the hair:

(a) temporary
(b) semi-permanent
(c) quasi-permanent
(d) permanent oxidation
(e) bleach
(f) henna or camomile.

3 Explain how a colourist can control the degree of lift achieved by the application of a bleach and give an example of when each of the following types of hair lighteners would be used:

(a) powder/paste
(b) emulsion
(c) oil
(d) lightening shampoo
(e) lightening setting lotion.

4 Explain why metallic dyes are not manufactured for professional use and how their use can limit a client's range of future hairdressing services.

Choosing a Colour

4.1 Client consultation

The discussion which takes place between you and a client before any hairdressing service is begun is called a *consultation*. This is when you and your client discuss, agree and confirm the course of action that will be taken to achieve the client's desired colour result by carrying out a colour analysis. You will need to ask plenty of questions during the consultation. There are many different types of questioning technique and the ones which are recommended can be distinguished as follows:

- Open questions
- Closed questions
- Probing questions.

Open questions are useful because they require the person being questioned to give information. Open questions begin with the words 'what', 'which', 'when', 'how', 'where', and 'why'. For example:

Q. 'When did you last have your highlights done?'
A. 'Around Christmas time.'

Closed questions are questions that have a 'yes' or 'no' answer and are useful for confirming points that have been raised. For example:

Q. 'So, you had these highlights about four months ago?'
A. 'Yes.'

Probing questions are used to investigate certain points in greater detail. For example:

Q. 'Tell me what you liked and didn't like about these highlights?'
A. 'Well, . . .'

You can see from these examples that it is useful to question in this sequence:

OPEN – CLOSED – PROBE

As well as questioning your client, you may find it helpful to use visual aids such as shade charts. Remember too, that the hair colour of colleagues can be used to show a client a particular colour or colouring technique. For example, 'So you like the colour of Mandy's hair? Let me call her over so that you can have a closer look at her highlights'.

Hair colour analysis can be divided into three main areas:

(1) The scalp;
(2) The hair;
(3) The client.

Each of these will be fully explained but for a quick reference see *Colour analysis – at a glance* (Fig. 4.1).

N.B. It is important to remember to carry out a test cutting first if you are unsure of what the colour result will be (see [2.5]).

4.2 Colour analysis – the scalp

Under certain conditions the use of hair colorants can cause severe irritation, allergic reaction or worsen existing scalp conditions. Always check the scalp thoroughly for any contra-indications before proceeding with a hair colour application.

Cuts/abrasions/sores
The product may cause severe discomfort to the client and worsen some conditions. If the cut or abrasion can be isolated, it may be possible to use a colorant, but the application must be careful and selective.

Infectious conditions
Under *no* circumstances should *any* hairdressing treatment be given if the client is suffering from an infectious condition such as impetigo, ringworm, lice, etc.

Cysts and warts

Normally cysts and warts do not restrict the use of hair colour, but if they are open or weeping, follow the same advice as given in (1).

Dandruff/dry scalp

The use of colorants can make the scalp drier. Dry scalps have a tendency to stain easily. If using a semi-permanent or tint, make sure your removal of the product at the basin is properly carried out to avoid this.

Oily scalp

An oily scalp does not affect the use of hair colour. Using tint or bleach on an oily scalp can counteract the activity of the sebaceous glands because they have a drying effect on the hair and skin.

4.3   Colour analysis – the hair

The quality of the hair you work with will affect the choice of product and application technique, and also the performance and durability of the colour you use.

The effect of condition

Porous hair will absorb colour easily because of the open cuticle. Temporary and semi-permanent colour may 'grab' and last longer than expected. Permanent colours, however, will fade more quickly because the colour molecules can escape via the open cuticle.

Resistant hair has a tightly closed cuticle, making it difficult for some products to work effectively. If using a permanent oxidation tint on very resistant white hair, try pre-softening the hair first to aid penetration of the product (see *Pre-softening resistant hair* [5.8]).

Internal damage to the hair may be increased by the further use of tints or pre-lighteners. If necessary, consider alternative means of colouring such hair.

N.B. *The condition of the external (cuticle) and internal (cortex) structure of hair can be assessed by performing porosity and elasticity tests. (See [2.1] and [2.2].)*

The effect of texture and density

The texture and the amount of hair on the head should not make too much difference to your colour choice, but *do* consider the following points:

- Very fine, highlights or lowlights will not show up well in a mass of curly hair;
- Too many highlights or lowlights in fine hair will give the appearance of a full colour application;
- If the hair is fine but dense (i.e. lots of fine hair) a full-head colour application will appear more intense (greater depth of tone) because you are seeing a greater quantity of coloured hair. This is particularly noticeable when using ash colours, because these also make the hair appear darker than it actually is.

The effect of previous chemical treatment

Perms and curl relaxers affect the internal structure of the hair and the cuticle. The hair will be drier than natural hair and more inclined to absorb colours quickly. Tints fade rapidly on hair which has been subjected to over-perming and frequent relaxing treatments.

If colour has been used on the hair, try to find out what the product was, as some react unfavourably with others. This is particularly important if the client coloured her or his hair at home. Trying to establish what products clients used at home takes time, and you will need to ask plenty of exploratory questions – for example:

'Was the product shampooed into the hair and left for a while?'
If yes, the product could have been semi-permanent or permanent.

'Were two things mixed together?'
If yes, this indicates it was a permanent quasi-permanent colour, since these types of products need mixing with an oxidant in order to work.

'How long did the packaging say it would last?'
'Until next shampoo' means temporary; 'for a few washes' means probably semi-permanent; 'gradual fade' could mean either semi-permanent or permanent; 'lasts and lasts' means permanent.

'Did the packaging say the product would lighten or brighten?'
If yes, it could be some type of bleach- or peroxide-based product.

'Does the colour gradually appear the more it was continually applied?'

If yes, this suggests the use of a progressive colorant.

N.B. Some home-products are referred to as 'shampoo-in' colorants. This can refer to the method of application rather than the lasting effect.

Do *not* proceed with a colour treatment unless you have established what has been used on the hair or have carried out all necessary precautionary tests.

The effect of white hair

The amount of white hair present is usually referred to as a percentage. For example, 50% white hair means that half the hair is white, while the other half is the client's natural colour. The amount of white hair may also be greater in some areas than others. This could influence your choice of product and appli-cation technique.

Temporary colorants cannot fully disguise white hair. Semi-permanent colorants can cover up to 30% white hair while a quasi-permanent (or cosmetic colorant) can cover up to 50%. Permanent oxidation tints can successfully cover hair which is 100% white but you must read the manufacturers' instructions because special colour mixes are sometimes necessary to ensure the result will not be too bright. If using a fashion shade for covering 50% white hair using either a quasi-permanent (or cosmetic colorant) or permanent oxidation tint, you will normally be instructed to mix equal parts of the fashion shade with the corresponding base shade. Remember that unattractive 'carrot' shades will be produced by applying henna to white hair.

Depth and tone

Depth describes how light or how dark the hair is and is measured on a scale between 1 or 2 (the darkest) to 10 or 11 (the lightest).

Tone refers to the colour we actually see. Words used to describe tone include copper, gold, red, burgundy, ash, mahogany and so on.

The depth and tone of colorants are shown on manufacturers' shade charts.

You will need to establish the depth of the client's natural hair in order to know if the product you intend using has the ability to achieve the target colour. To determine the depth of the client's natural hair colour, first ensure that he or she is positioned in a good light so that you can see the true hair colour. Daylight is best for this but 'warm white' fluorescent tube lighting closely simulates natural daylight. As natural hair colour varies over the head and is often darker or lighter in some areas, divide the hair down the centre from forehead to nape. By doing this, you will be able to see any variation of depth and the distribution of white hair. Examine the hair and classify how light or how dark it is on the depth scale. All manufacturers' shade charts for oxidation tints contain natural depth colours, so referring to one of these charts will help you confirm your judgement of the depth, by making a comparison. If the hair has already been tinted or pre-lightened, you need to establish the depth of *both* the regrowth and the previously coloured hair.

The tone of the natural hair is also important to you. If it is golden, copper or red, it will be more difficult to pre-lighten, and this natural warmth can also interfere with the final colour result. The tone can also be described by the use of numbers or letters – so check manufacturers' information and shade charts so that you know how each tone is described.

4.4 Colour analysis – the client

Just as a hairstyle should suit your client, so should the colour. Colour is used for different reasons and to create various effects, but it still must suit your client's appearance and personality.

The client will often use words in a different way to the hairdresser; their idea of 'red hair' may be totally different to your idea of 'red hair'. Therefore use plenty of aids such as shade charts and pictures.

Explain the advantages of having hair colour along with any commitments the client will need to make. The type of product you intend using and the application technique should suit the client's life-style and pocket. A busy client may not have the time to visit the salon for regular regrowth applications. Other clients may prefer a larger initial expenditure with fewer subsequent visits (e.g. weave highlights).

Listed below are some points for you to consider.

Why does the client want colour?
– to cover white hair?

  – to match regrowth to lengths and ends?
  – to make him or her look more youthful?
  – to lighten the hair?
  – for a change?
  – to darken the hair?

Sometimes, husbands, wives, boyfriends or girlfriends have persuaded the client to have a colour which may not be suitable. Talk to the client, question the reasons for the colour choice and offer other suggestions. Consider the following factors:

Age
Over the age of 35, recommend a colour no darker than the client's natural hair colour.

Skin colour
Flushed or ruddy complexions will look redder if red hair colours are used. Pale complexions will look paler if very dark colours are used.

Eye colour
If possible, match the hair colour to the eyes to emphasize them and make them look larger.

Personality
Generally speaking, the more introvert the client is, the more subtle the colour should be. The more extrovert, the more adventurous you can be!

Favourite colours
If a client wears one colour a lot, try to complement this with an appropriate hair colour.

Time and cost
Permanent, all-over hair colours require a firm commitment on the part of the client. Can he or she spare 2–3 hours in the salon every month for a regrowth application? If not, suggest partial colouring techniques or highlights. A client may think that the cost of weave highlights in her long hair is expensive, so explain that she will not need to revisit the salon for another four to six months for more colour applications. A £60 outlay to last six months for the weave highlights could therefore be cheaper than four or five visits for tinting regrowth at £20 a visit – and it will save valuable time.

You *sell* the client your service.

None of the points mentioned, (the scalp, the hair, the client) can be considered in isolation. They all form part of the analysis. Remember that the client comes to you for professional advice, and you should offer this in an authoritative but pleasant manner. Many clients will also need reassuring about having hair colour.

4.5　Colour analysis – at a glance

There are many different factors to be taken into consideration when analysing hair prior to colouring. Fig. 4.1 condenses this information into a list of important details to be covered. With experience, the sequence of colour analysis will become second nature.

4.6　Manufacturers' shade charts

Manufacturers produce shade charts for their colorants, which have hair samples (usually synthetic), showing the colour range available. Shade charts are generally supplied free to salons on the initial purchase of the products. The samples may be enclosed in a type of folder, on a display card, or attached to a type of key ring.

The samples are usually made from white nylon which has been coloured with the product, so that they take on the 'true' colour. Natural tones in hair interfere with colour results. Make sure that your colour analysis is thorough and that you know the capabilities of the hair product range in the salon.

Because shade charts are primarily for showing clients the available shades, they are usually presented in an appealing way, with photographs, etc. The shades are given appealing names. Have you ever tried giving clients the chart upside down? Although they are supposed to be looking at the *colours*, they also want to see the *name* of the colour they have chosen. Manufacturers realize how much we are influenced by the names and so spend time and money researching what names would be most appealing at that time. This is why colours (especially tints) are given a name *and* a number. We don't usually talk to our clients using the numbering system! The names are for using with our client and the numbers are for us the hairdressers, because they tell us *exactly* what depth and tone a colour is.

When a client comes into the salon and asks, for instance, to be the colour of a Red Setter dog, do you presume you are both talking about the same colour? A shade chart can help prevent

COLOUR ANALYSIS QUESTIONNAIRE
(to be stapled to client's record card)

Client name: _____ Colourist: _____ Date:_____

The scalp

Any cuts, abrasions or sores present? _____

Any sign of infection or disease? _____

Any cysts or warts? _____

Any other conditions e.g. dandruff? _____

Comments about health of scalp: _____

_____

_____

The hair

What condition? _____

What texture and density? _____

What previous chemical services? _____

Percentage of white hair? _____

White hair evenly distributed? _____

Natural depth? _____

Is natural tone warm? _____

The client

Reason for coloration? _____

Approx. age group? _____

Skin tone? _____

Eye colour? _____

Client's favourite colours? _____

Any comments? _____

_____

Target colour: _____

Products to be used: _____

Application technique: _____

Strength of hydrogen peroxide to be used: _____

Expected development time: Roots: _____ Lengths and ends: _____

Fig. 4.1 Colour analysis – at a glance.

misunderstandings. By consulting the chart, both you and the client can point to the colour you imagine a Red Setter to be.

4.7 Colouring number systems

Manufacturers use an International Colour Code (ICC) system to describe the shades they produce. These numbers tell the hairdresser exactly what depth and tone the artificial colour has.

Depth

This describes how light or how dark the colour is. Depth ranges on a scale between 1 or 2 (the darkest) and 10 or 11 (the lightest). Remember that white hair has no depth or tone because technically it is colourless.

    2/0   black
    3/0   dark brown
    4/0   medium brown
    5/0   light brown
    6/0   dark blonde
    7/0   medium blonde
    8/0   light blonde
    9/0   very light blonde
    10/0 extra light blonde
    11/0 high-lift blonde shades

Therefore, a client with natural dark blonde hair is described as having a natural base shade (depth) of 6/0.

Tone

Tone describes the colour we actually see. It may be golden, ash, copper, etc. The number used to specify the tone always follows a dot or an oblique.

    /1   blue ash
    /2   mauve ash
    /3   gold (yellow)
    /4   copper (orange)
    /5   burgundy or mahogany
    /6   red

Therefore, a colour which has the number 6/1 tells you it has the depth of dark blonde and has an ash tone; that is dark ash blonde.

What is 9/3?
What is 7/3?

Sometimes, manufacturers use letters instead of numbers to describe the tones of permanent colorants. For example, R = red, G = gold, A = ash, C = copper and so on.

You may come across two numbers being used to describe the tone of a colour. The first number nearest the oblique stroke is the main or primary tone. The second number is the underlying or secondary tone. Here are some examples:

8/34   Depth = light blonde. The primary tone is gold with a delicate back-up tone of copper.
8/43   Depth = light blonde. This time, the primary tone is copper with a delicate back-up tone of gold.
8/44   Depth = light blonde. The use of the same number twice indicates that the primary tone of copper is intensified by the addition of the same colour as the secondary tone.
7/03   Depth = medium blonde. This has no primary tone and the secondary tone is gold. Therefore, 7/03 contains less gold tones than 7/3.

Fig. 4.2 is an example of how the numbers on a permanent oxidation tint shade chart may appear. Remember that the intermixing of the available colours means that you can blend an almost infinite range of colours to suit your clients.

4.8   Choosing the correct permanent oxidation tint

There are two main factors which will influence your product selection and the final colour result:

(1)   The client's natural base;
(2)   The depth and tone of the target colour.

The client's natural base

For hair which is over 50% white *either* pre-soften first to ensure complete coverage *or* choose a colour which contains no primary

Tone Depth	Basic Shades	/1 Blue Ash	/2 Mauve Ash	/3 Golden	/4 Copper	/5 Mahogany	/6 Red
11 High-lift Blondes	11/0	11/1	11/2	11/03			
10 Extra light Blonde	10/0	10/1	10/21	10/03			
9 Very Light Blonde	9/0	9/1 9/01		9/3 9/03	9/04		
8 Light Blonde	8/0	8/1 8/01		8/3 8/03 8/34	8/43 8/44		
7 Medium Blonde	7/0	7/1 7/01	7/2	7/3 7/03	7/4 7/43		
6 Dark Blonde	6/0	6/1			6/43	6/52	6/6 6/62
5 Light Brown	5/0		5/2	5/3			
4 Medium Brown	4/0		4/26		4/4	4/52	
3 Dark Brown	3/0						3/6
2 Black	2/0						

light → (top, Depth axis) / Depth / Dark ↓

Fig. 4.2 Example of numbering system on a shade chart.

tone. (Fashion shades will produce intense or very bright results on hair with over 50% white.)

Examples:

Natural base – 5/0 (60% white)
Target colour – 6/1
Selected colour – 6/01

Manufacturers produce tints especially for use on hair which contains a high percentage of white. These tints contain extra base shade that will help replace the pigment which is lost when hair turns white and will prevent the tone from being too intense in the final result. You can recognize these tints by their number, as they will always have a naught after the point or oblique stroke, telling you that the primary tone is replaced with extra base shade – for example, 7/01.

If the natural base contains warmth remember that this will affect the final result – that is, it will be redder or more golden than expected.

When you are assessing the depth of the client's natural hair colour during the analysis, you only have to see a glint of red, gold or copper to know that the hair contains warmth. Obviously, a client with a natural head of red hair has a much warmer natural base than a client with just a hint of gold, but it is important to be aware of how the warmth present in natural hair affects the final result. If warmth is not required, some of the natural warm pigment can be cancelled by using a colour which contains ash. The ash tone will help to kill the excess warmth, preventing results which are more golden, copper or red than desired.

Examples:

Natural base – 6/0 (contains warmth)
Target colour – 7/0
Selected colour – 7/1

The depth and tone of target colour

If tints were capable of achieving high degrees of lift on all natural colours, there would be no need for pre-lightener. The darker the natural base, the harder it is for the tint to lighten the natural colour.

Many manufacturers now produce special lightening tints, which have the power to make the hair lighter than normal tints. The choice of hydrogen peroxide strength is the main way of ensuring that enough lift will be achieved when using normal tints. However, if you increase the hydrogen peroxide strength to greater than that recommended by the product manufacturers, you will not get the true target colour. This is because the tones contained in tints are extremely well-balanced and delicate. Too strong a peroxide will kill the tone.

For normal tints, 20 or 30 vol hydrogen peroxide is normally used:

20 vol – for 1-2 shades of lift
30 vol – for maximum lift (up to 3 shades)

Examples:

Natural Base – 6/0
Target colour – 9/1
Selected colour – 9/1 + 30 vols

Natural base – 5/0
Target colour – 7/31
Selected colour – 7/31 + 20 vols

Natural base – 3/0
Target colour – 4/45
Selected colour – 4/45 + 20 vols

N.B. The strength of hydrogen peroxide to be used will be stated in the manufacturers' instructions.

4.9   Customized colour mixes

Once you are familiar with manufacturers' numbering systems, you will be able to intermix colours, increasing your ability to create personalized shades for your clients. This knowledge of intermixing will also be helpful if you find that a particular colour you need is out of stock. Please note, that colours should only be intermixed from the same manufacturer's colour range.

Examples:

half 7/2 + half 5/2 = 6/2
half 10/1 + half 8/1 = 9/1
half 4/0 + half 6/0 = 5/0

What would the following mixes make?

half 7/3   + half 5/3   =
half 6/43 + half 8/43 =
half 6/52 + half 4/52 =

There are some shades which should *not* be intermixed and these are shown in Fig. 4.3. Many manufacturers also produce a range of special 'mix-tones' which are added in small quantities to increase the tones of a particular colour. They are concentrated colours available in cream and liquid form. These mix-tone colours are strong and are usually added in small quantities – one to six capfuls if they are liquid and perhaps 5–30 cm if in cream form and being squeezed out of a tube. For example, to increase the golden tone for the target colour of 8/3, you could add some 0/33 (gold) mix-tone. You will have noticed that the number used to describe mix-tones has a zero indicating that the colour has no depth, only tone.

Unsuitable mix	Reason
half 9/04 + half 9/1	The ash (/1) will neutralize the delicate copper (/04) tone.
half 7/2 + half 7/3	The mauve (/2) will neutralize the gold (/3).
half 8/03 + half 8/0	The delicate golden secondary tone (/03) will be lost.
half 4/0 + half 5/0	Is the colourist unsure about which colour to apply?
half 4/52 + half 8/44	Neither the depths nor tones correspond with each other.
half 10/1 + half 6/1	Is the colourist unsure of what depth they are aiming for?

Fig. 4.3 Unsuitable intermixing of permanent oxidation colorants.

4.10 Bleach bases for toners

When the natural base is too dark for the target colour, it is necessary to pre-lighten the hair and then apply a toner. It is *very* important that toners are applied to the correct bleach base (see Fig. 3.7). If this is not done, the toner will not achieve the target colour. Bleaching lightens hair by first eliminating the black/brown pigment, then the red pigment and finally the yellow pigment. The bleaching product is rinsed from the hair when the desired amount of pigment has been eliminated – in other words, when the correct bleach base has been achieved so that it can act as the 'undercoat' for the toner.

Note that it is impossible to bleach hair lighter than very pale yellow because keratin itself is pale yellow. We can create the *illusion* of white hair by lifting the hair to very pale yellow and then applying a pale pastel toner to subdue the unwanted yellow tones.

Examples:

Target colour: 7/43
Natural base: 3
Bleach base: orange

Target colour: 6/62
Natural base: 3
Bleach base: reddish/orange

Target colour: 10/1
Natural base: 5
Bleach base: very pale yellow

The above examples show how the bleach bases must complement the tone of the target colour to serve as the correct undercoat.

What would be the ideal bleach bases for the following target colours?

Target colour: 9
Natural base: 4

Target colour: 8/1
Natural base: 3

4.11 Colouring Afro-type hair

Many salons fear colouring Afro-type hair because to them, it is an unknown quantity. The pigment in Afro-type hair is very dense, making the use of pre-lighteners necessary to create any noticeable change in the colour depth. However, because Afro-type hair has probably been relaxed or permed, extra care and precautionary measures will need to be taken. Natural Afro hair will not be as fragile as chemically treated hair so, basically, colouring processes will be the same for this type as European hair, with equally stunning results.

What precautions should be taken if colouring permed or relaxed Afro-type hair?

Perming and relaxing affects the internal structure of the hair, making the hair fragile because it loses some of its strength and elasticity. Some clients have certain areas of their hair relaxed more than others, so to create specific looks it is important to question the client to find out as much as you can. Hair that has been relaxed to a major extent should be treated with great care. A test cutting is *essential*, taking hair samples from several areas if necessary. Tints and pre-lighteners for colouring all the hair should be avoided to prevent further damage. Partial colouring, such as highlighting and touch colouring, using low peroxide strength, can be carried out provided a test cutting has been done first, to check colour product performance and results, Extensive damage could be caused by applying tint or bleach immediately over hair which has just been permed or relaxed. Allow at least two deep conditioning treatments to take place before applying colour. This will help to remoisturize the hair, preparing it for further chemical processing.

What type of colouring techniques and products are recommended for Afro-type hair?

Henna has been very popular in many salons, though its main function was as a conditioning product rather than a colorant. As the pigment in Afro-type hair is very dense, henna has no dramatic effect in changing the colour.

Afro-type hair which has been chemically processed by perming or relaxing will obviously be more porous than natural Afro hair. Because of the hair's increased receptivity to colour products when it is porous, semi-permanent colours can work particularly well. Of course, brighter, richer colours should be chosen to make any significant difference.

Temporary colours can be used to create exciting, fashionable looks on any hair type.

4.12 Revision questions

1 What are the three main areas of hair colour analysis?

2 What is meant by the term *target colour*?

3 What does the word *depth* describe?

4 What does the word *tone* describe?

5 If the client's natural base is *warm*, what considerations will you need to make in the choice of colour to be applied?

6 What does ICC stand for?

7 In manufacturers' colour code numbers, what does the number *before* the oblique stroke or point tell you about a colour?

8 What does the number (or numbers) *after* the oblique stroke or point tell you about a colour?

9 On what natural bases would you use a high-lift tint?

10 When would you use special mix-tone colorants?

11 What is meant by the term *regrowth*?

12 What is the lightest that hair can be bleached?

4.13 Advanced questions

1 Explain the importance of producing the correct bleach base for toners and describe the various degrees of lightness which hair goes through during bleaching.

2 Explain the importance of a full client consultation before a hair colouring service and describe how you would do this.

3 Explain why colours may appear more intense on abundant, fine hair as opposed to coarse, sparse hair.

4 Describe the purpose of pre-softening and the effect it has on hair structure.

5

Preparation of the Hair and Colouring Products

Always read the manufacturers' instructions to find out how the hair should be prepared for the application of colorants.

Product manufacturers test the products in their own laboratories to assess and evaluate the best circumstances for product performance. If a product is designed to be applied to towel-dried hair *only*, for instance, there is obviously a reason for this so take note of the instructions.

It should be remembered that a hairdresser can be sued if proven to be negligent. Certain products such as tints and bleaches *must not* be applied to any area where there is broken skin. If you ignore the instructions written by the manufacturer about such dangers and it results in a client taking you to court, you will have no defence.

5.1 Temporary colorants

Temporary colorants are applied either to clean, damp hair or to finished styles, so read the manufacturers' instructions. Temporary colours in the form of mousses and rinses are applied to hair after shampooing. The hair should be towel-dried or the colour will be diluted by the excess moisture left in the hair. An average head of hair can hold up to 60 ml of moisture before dripping! Gels, sprays and paints are normally applied to the hair when the style is finished. Be careful not to apply too much colour – it is very easy to get carried away!

5.2 Semi-permanent colorants

Semi-permanent colorants are applied to hair which has been shampooed and towel-dried. Applying conditioners before a semi-permanent is not recommended unless the hair is very porous, because conditioners can create a barrier on the hair shaft, making it difficult for the product to penetrate. The action of shampooing makes the hair more receptive to the semi-permanent colour because it opens the cuticle slightly and removes any sebum which would act as a barrier. Some semi-permanents must be applied to freshly shampooed hair that has been thoroughly dried, so check the instructions.

5.3 Quasi-permanent or cosmetic colorants

Quasi-permanent (or cosmetic) colorants are either applied like a shampoo to freshly shampooed, towel-dried hair or to dry hair, so it is important to read the manufacturers' instructions. Usually, if you are applying the colorant for the first time, you will apply it like a shampoo to damp hair from an applicator flask or bottle. If it is a subsequent application to cover a regrowth, or if the hair is porous and you want to avoid colour build-up on the lengths and ends, the hair may not need to be shampooed and the colorant is applied to dry, unwashed hair – but check the instructions.

5.4 Permanent oxidation colorants

Permanent oxidation colorants are applied to *unwashed* hair. The action of shampooing stimulates the scalp and removes sebum. Products such as tints will irritate the scalp more if the protective barrier of sebum has been removed. Afro-type hair which has been relaxed or permed may be coated with moisturizing products such as gloss creams and curl activators. If the application of these is heavy, you will need to shampoo first. In this case, give *one gentle* shampoo, and then thoroughly dry the hair.

Be careful when brushing the hair before applying a permanent colour. It is easy to scratch the scalp by harsh brushing, making the tint feel uncomfortable for the client when it is applied.

Always check for cuts and abrasions on the scalp before a tint application. Tint should *not* be applied to any area where there is a break in the skin's surface, because this would cause severe discomfort. Cover any cuts and abrasions with a barrier cream and avoid the area completely.

Some salons apply barrier cream to the hairline and ears before applying a tint. This is not necessary if your application is careful, as we are in the business of colouring hair and not skin! There is also a risk that the barrier cream may accidentally get onto the hair, forming an impenetrable coating on the hair shaft.

5.5   Bleach

Bleach is applied to *unwashed* hair to avoid undue irritation of the scalp. Shampooing is not necessary before the application unless the hair is particularly oily. If you do need to shampoo first, just give *one gentle* shampoo and then thoroughly dry the hair.

Lightening shampoos (or bleach baths) and lightening setting lotions are applied to shampooed hair which has been towel-dried.

5.6   Henna

Henna is applied to shampooed, towel-dried hair. The action of the shampoo opens the cuticle and removes any sebum which would act as a barrier. If a client has shampooed their hair the day before the appointment, give one quick shampoo to remove sebum and products such as hairspray from the hair.

5.7   Camomile

Camomile, like henna, is applied to freshly shampooed hair which has been towel-dried.

5.8   Pre-softening resistant hair

What does pre-softening mean?

Pre-softening makes hair more porous (raises the cuticle) by applying peroxide and then drying under a warm drier.

What type of hair needs pre-softening?

Hair that is resistant to tints needs pre-softening. A porosity test will enable you to assess whether the cuticle scales are open or closed; if the hair feels smooth and glossy you can presume that the hair could resist the tint. White hair can be particularly resistant. Complete coverage by a tint on resistant white hair would be impossible, without pre-softening first.

When is pre-softening necessary?

- When you are not achieving good tint coverage on white hair.
- When you are doing a virgin tint application on hair that is white, or partially white, and the target shade is lighter than the natural shade.

- When you are doing a virgin tint application on hair that is white, or partially white, and the target shade is darker than the natural shade.

Procedure

Hair with a regrowth

- Apply liquid hydrogen peroxide (20 or 30 vol) to the regrowth area prior to the root retouch application.
- Dry the hair under a drier.
- Proceed with the tint application as normal.

Virgin hair going lighter

- Apply liquid hydrogen peroxide (30 vol) to the lengths and ends only.
- Dry the peroxide into the hair under a warm drier.
- Apply tint to root area.
- Immediately proceed with tint application to lengths and ends.
- Develop tint according to manufacturers' instructions.

Virgin hair going darker (pre-softening is necessary only if the hair contains white)

- Apply liquid hydrogen peroxide (20 or 30 vol) to the white hair.
- Dry the peroxide into the hair under a warm drier.
- Apply tint to root area.
- Immediately proceed with tint application to lengths and ends.
- Develop tint according to manufacturers' instructions.

Pre-softening is the most efficient technique for preparing hair for a virgin tint application. The conventional method (see virgin bleach application) is very time-consuming and requires a larger amount of product.

If there is a large amount of white hair present, apply the hydrogen peroxide to this area first.

5.9 Preparation of temporary colorants

Are temporary colorants ready for use?

Yes, all except the concentrated liquids. However, always shake the container, if recommended by the manufacturers, as sometimes the actual colouring agent settles at the bottom of the can or bottle.

Can you mix temporary colorants together?

Yes, as long as they are of the same consistency, and are mixed before applying. It would be impossible to blend together a liquid and gel *or* mousse and spray. There are so many temporary colours to choose from that mixing is not normally necessary.

There is, of course, nothing to stop you from using more than one type on the hair, such as a spray and crayons, or indeed, using more than one colour on the same head of hair.

How are concentrated temporary colorants prepared?

These can either be added to setting lotions or mixed with warm water (warm water helps the colour mix more easily). There are instructions to help you with the correct dilution, which is normally measured in drops. Really vibrant colours can be achieved by using a lot of the concentrate or by adding to an already coloured setting lotion. For example, to make copper setting lotion brighter, add a few drops of a red or copper concentrate.

Always remember that if the hair is porous, the colours could 'grab' and last longer than one shampoo. If in doubt of the colour result, try the colour on a few strands before applying it over the whole head.

5.10 Preparation of semi-permanent colorants

Are semi-permanents ready for use?

Yes. Always shake the container before use if recommended by the manufacturer.

Can you mix semi-permanents together?

Yes. If using more than one colour, blend them together in a bowl before applying. However, this is difficult if the product comes in a mousse form, and is *not* recommended.

Remember that some semi-permanents contain small amounts of para-compounds, chemicals which can cause an allergic reaction on some people. Read the packaging to see if a skin test is necessary.

Also, don't forget that if the hair is porous, the colour could 'grab' and last longer than expected. Do a test cutting if in doubt of the colour result.

5.11 Preparation of quasi-permanent or cosmetic colorants

Are quasi-permanent or cosmetic colorants ready for use?

No. Quasi-permanent (or cosmetic) colorants need to be mixed with an oxidant (hydrogen peroxide) before they are applied to the hair. The hydrogen peroxide added to this type of colorant is relatively low in strength (up to 3% or 10 vol) and may be called a 'colour releaser', 'colour activator' or 'colour developer'. Usually, the colorant is mixed at a ratio of 2:1. This means that two parts of oxidant are used to one part of the colorant. As an example, you might be instructed to mix 40 ml of the oxidant with 20 ml of the colorant.

Can you mix quasi-permanent or cosmetic colorants together?

Yes. Some manufacturers produce special red, orange and purple mix-tones in their range of quasi-permanent or cosmetic colorants to intensify colour results.

5.12 Preparation of permanent oxidation colorants

Are permanent colorants (tints) ready for use?

No. They are always mixed with hydrogen peroxide. The amount of peroxide will often depend on the product being used so *always check manufacturers' instructions*. The majority of tints are mixed with equal parts of peroxide – for example 60 ml tint plus 60 ml peroxide.

Most tubes are marked to tell you when you have squeezed out one-quarter, one-half or three-quarters of the product. Always squeeze the tube at the bottom – it helps to avoid wastage. There are special keys available to help you get accurate measurements.

Bottle tints do not usually have markings on the outside, but the amount of product it holds will be printed on the label. Tint bottles are usually dark to protect the contents from becoming affected by light, so it is tricky to get an accurate reading if you only want to pour out one-quarter or one-half of the tint in the bottle. Pouring the tint into a measure is by far the most accurate method.

If you are using the whole bottle of tint, simply empty the contents into a bowl and then refill the bottle with hydrogen peroxide to give you the correct amount. Check manufacturers' instructions however: usually the amount of peroxide is the same as the amount of tint.

When using a measure, taking a reading by standing above the measure will give you a false reading. To get an accurate reading, hold the measure at eye level or better still, place it on a shelf level with your eyes (Fig. 5.1).

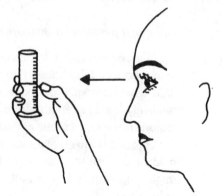

Fig. 5.1 Taking a correct reading from a measure.

How do you mix a tint?

- Measure the amount of tint required and put into a non-metallic bowl (Fig. 5.2). (Metal reacts unfavourably with tint and peroxide.)
- If using more than one colour, blend these together with your brush.
- Measure the amount of hydrogen peroxide required for the amount of tint you have in your bowl.
- Gradually stir the peroxide into the tint until they are completely blended together.
- Allow the tint to stand for a couple of minutes before use to allow the mixture to stabilize.

5.13 Preparation of bleaches

Are bleaches ready for use?

No. They are mixed with hydrogen peroxide and sometimes other ingredients such as special boosters (or controllers) and oils (or gels). Manufacturers' instructions should always be followed.

How do you mix a bleach?

Powder (paste)
Powders and pastes should be mixed to the correct consistency by

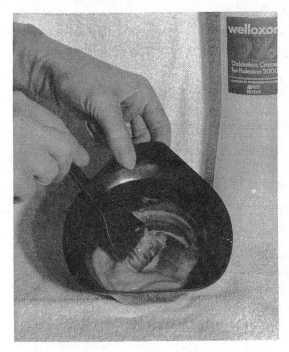

Fig. 5.2 Mixing a tint.

following manufacturers' instructions. Liquid or cream peroxide can be used.

Oil
This is normally mixed with equal parts of cream or liquid peroxide.

Emulsion
The mixture consists of cream or liquid peroxide, boosters/controllers and a special oil/gel. The number of boosters/controllers needed will depend on how many shades of lift you require. The strength of peroxide is dictated by how difficult the hair is to lighten (if it is dark or contains warmth).

Lightening shampoo
A lightening shampoo (or bleach bath) is prepared by mixing the following ingredients:

1 part 6% (20 vol) hydrogen peroxide
1 part powder or paste bleach
1 part shampoo
1 part water

Lightening setting lotion

Lightening setting lotions require no preparation because they are produced ready to be applied to hair.

5.14 Preparation of henna

Is henna ready for use?

No. It comes in powder form which needs to be mixed with very hot water to make a thick paste.

What can be added to the henna paste to improve its conditioning or colouring properties?

Many salons add ingredients such as egg yolk to help improve the consistency of the henna paste and help make the hair shine. Adding acetic acid will make the final result browner, red wine will result in a more red result and black coffee will help darken the hair.

5.15 Preparation of camomile

Is camomile ready for use?

No. There are two methods of preparing camomile:

Method 1. Pour boiling water on the dried camomile flower heads and allow the solution to 'brew' like you would tea. Once cooled, the solution can be poured through the hair as a rinse.

Method 2. Dried camomile flower heads are crushed with kaolin then mixed with very hot water to form a paste like henna.

5.16 Hydrogen peroxide

Hydrogen peroxide is the most common chemical used in hairdressing to provide oxygen. It is used to lighten the natural pigment of the hair and to develop the colour of oxidation tints.

Chemically, hydrogen peroxide is similar in structure to water, except that it has an extra oxygen which is loosely attached.

$$H_2O \qquad H_2O_2$$
$$\text{water} \qquad \text{hydrogen peroxide}$$

How do I measure hydrogen peroxide strength?

If ever you look at a hydrogen peroxide container it will say one of two things – volume or percentage strength. Most of us use the peroxide without knowing what these mean; although we know that 40 vol is twice as strong as 20 vol, and 12% is twice as strong as 6%.

Volume strength is the number of parts of free oxygen that can be given off by one part of hydrogen peroxide if it completely decomposes. For example, a gallon container of 20 vol hydrogen peroxide could give off 20 gallons of oxygen. A gallon of 40 vol hydrogen peroxide could give off 40 gallons of oxygen; it is twice as strong because it can give off twice as much oxygen.

Percentage strength is a more chemical concept. It is actually saying how many parts of pure hydrogen peroxide are found in every 100 parts of the peroxide solution. 6% peroxide contains 6 g of peroxide in every 100 g of solution, while 12% peroxide contains 12 g of peroxide in every 100 g of solution. Because 12% peroxide contains twice as much peroxide as 6%, it is twice as strong.

If you are used to working with one particular strength of peroxide and suddenly find yourself faced with the other sort, it is a simple matter to convert to the one you are familiar with. Just remember that *3% is equal to 10 vol*. Now look at the following section on conversion and work through the examples.

5.17 Converting hydrogen peroxide strengths

These conversions of hydrogen peroxide strengths are easy to do once you have mastered the method. Remember the key fact that 3% = 10 vol. If ever you are asked to convert something in the salon, the numbers that you use will always be divisible by 3 if they are percentage strengths, or divisible by 10 if they are volume strengths.

Volume to percentage

To convert from volume to percentage, you simply divide by 10 (cross off a zero) and multiply by 3.

What you are doing is finding out how many tens are in the number because, when you convert it, it will have that number of threes. Without looking at the answers, which are given below, try to work the following to percentages strengths:

(a) 20 vol   (b) 40 vol   (c) 70 vol   (d) 100 vol

Percentage to volume

To convert percentage to volume, you simply divide by three and multiply by ten (add a zero).

What you are doing is finding out how many threes are in the number, because, when you convert it, it will have that number of tens. Without looking at the answers which are given below, try to convert the following to volume strengths:

(e) 9%   (f) 15%   (g) 21%   (h) 30%

How do I check hydrogen peroxide strength?

There is a special type of hydrometer available called a *peroxometer*. The stronger the hydrogen peroxide is, the denser it is when compared to water. The measurement of how dense a liquid is when compared to water is known as *relative density*. An older term, which means the same thing, is *specific gravity*.

The peroxometer is placed in the peroxide to be tested, which has usually been put in a transparent measuring cylinder that was supplied with the peroxometer. Allow the peroxometer to settle, tapping it if there are a lot of air bubbles on it. Now, if you hold the cylinder up to your eye and look you will see that the liquid level is against a number on the peroxometer scale. This is the strength of the peroxide. In Fig. 5.3 the volume strength shown is 70. Peroxometers are also available in percentage strength.

If you were to put a peroxometer into water, it would give off a reading of 0, as there is no oxygen left to give off.

It is good practice to test peroxide when it is delivered to the salon, or if it has been on the shelf a long time. I know of an incident where peroxide was mislabelled, so that what should have been 20 vol was in fact nearly 100 vol. If something containing peroxide does not seem to be working as fast as it should, check the strength in case it has started to deteriorate.

Cream peroxides cannot be checked for strength with a peroxometer. This is because they have been thickened up and contain added conditioner.

Answers:
(e) 9%   (b) 12%   (c) 21%   (d) 30%   (e) 30 vol   (f) 50 vol
(g) 70 vol   (h) 100 vol.

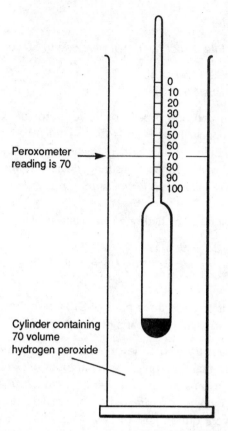

Peroxometer
reading is 70 →

0
10
20
30
40
50
60
70
80
90
100

Cylinder containing
70 volume
hydrogen peroxide

Fig. 5.3 Checking hydrogen peroxide strength.

How do I dilute hydrogen peroxide?

Liquid hydrogen peroxide (but not cream) can be diluted with water. This should ideally be distilled or deionized water, as tap water could cause the peroxide to start to decompose (because tap water is often slightly alkaline).

To dilute peroxide use the following formula:

A − B = C (cross a 0 off each number to make the working out easier).

The answer will be: B parts of peroxide to C parts of water.

A represents your stock strength of peroxide, while B represents the strength of the peroxide that you require. This formula can be used for either volume or percentage strengths. Here are two worked examples:

Examples:

(a) *Dilute 90 vol hydrogen peroxide to 50 vol.*

$$90 - 50 = 40$$
Answer: 5:4

Thus, if you add 5 parts of 90 vol peroxide to 4 parts of distilled water you will get 9 parts (5 + 4) of 50 vol peroxide. The word 'part' could be any kind of measure you have in the salon – a glass, bowl, cup or measuring device. *Whatever you use, make sure you only use it for measuring peroxide.*

(b) Dilute 21% hydrogen peroxide to 9%.

$$21 - 9 = 12$$
Answer: 9:12 or, since both of these can be divided by 3, 3:4

Thus, if you add three parts of 21% peroxide to 4 parts of distilled water you will get 7 parts of 9% peroxide.

Always try to get the smallest answer you can – it helps if you want to make up only a small amount of peroxide.

Try to answer the following questions yourself – the answers given below are expressed as the smallest numbers you can get. If you work out an answer as 2:4, the answer you will see given is 1:2, because both numbers can be divided by 2. You only make the answer you get smaller if *both* numbers can be divided by the same number.

Dilute the following:

(a) 90 vol to 70 vol   (b) 60 vol to 30 vol
(c) 60 vol to 20 vol   (d) 40 vol to 20 vol
(e) 18% to 9%   (f) 9% to 6%
(g) 12% to 20 vol (Hint: look at conversions and convert one number to proceed – both numbers must be either percentage or volume to dilute.)

What makes hydrogen peroxide decompose (lose its strength)?

There are three main things that make hydrogen peroxide go off – dust, alkalis and sunlight.

To avoid dust, always keep containers tightly closed, and replace lids as soon as possible. Measure the amount of peroxide you want to use. Do not pour any left-over peroxide back into the main container; it could have picked up dust and this could result in the loss of strength through the release of oxygen. If a container of peroxide has distorted sides, it is because it has released some of its oxygen, so open it slowly at arm's length.

Hydrogen peroxide is stable when it is acid, and stabilized peroxide has had acid added to it. Most of us have had the white burns of peroxide on our skin. If ever you do get hydrogen peroxide, or any hairdressing chemical on your skin, wash it off immediately with water until it stops stinging. Usually, we make hydrogen peroxide give off its oxygen by mixing it with an alkali, such as ammonium hydroxide or tint. One reason for not diluting peroxide with tap water is that it is often alkaline. This would not matter if the diluted peroxide were to be used quickly, but if it were stored the container could explode.

When you buy liquid hydrogen peroxide, it is usually in a white plastic container which is opaque – it does not allow light to pass through it. This stops the peroxide from going off too quickly. Even if you have such containers, do not leave them in direct light in case they heat up. Many of you may have seen brown glass bottles of peroxide, but these are going out of use because of possible accidents if the glass breaks.

> As hydrogen peroxide gives off oxygen, which supports combustion (fire), never store it next to flammable chemicals such as hairspray or setting lotion.

> Because damage caused by oxidation to hair can be severe, it is often recommended that anti-oxidant rinses are used. As the name implies, they stop oxidation and also close the cuticle. This can be important, because washing the product from the hair may not be enough to prevent creeping oxidation (the term used for oxidation caused by product retained in the hair after washing, of which you are unaware).

5.18   Revision questions

1   Why should harsh brushing be avoided before a whole head tint or bleach application?
2   What is the procedure if a cut or abrasion is found when examining the scalp prior to a tint or bleach application?
3   Why are tints and bleaches applied to unwashed hair?
4   How does pre-softening affect the hair shaft and when is it necessary?
5   What ingredients can be added to a henna mixture to boost the colour or improve the hair's shine?
6   In what circumstances would you use 20 and 30 vol hydrogen peroxide to develop a tint?
7   What is the best method of ensuring an accurate reading when using a measuring cylinder?
8   What are the differences between volume and percentage strengths of hydrogen peroxide?
9   How would you dilute 60 vol hydrogen peroxide to 30 vol? What type of water would you use and why?
10   Where and how should you store hydrogen peroxide? Give reasons.

5.19 Advanced questions

1   Explain why hydrogen peroxide needs to be stabilized and what is meant by *percentage* and *volume* strength.
2   Explain the importance of mixing hair colorants and preparing the hair to be coloured according to the manufacturers' instructions and state why colorants from different manufacturer product ranges should not be intermixed.
3   State when you would need to pre-soften hair and describe the procedure to be followed.
4   Describe how hydrogen peroxide should be stored and diluted.

6

Application of
Hair Colour

Colour application varies according to:

- The product being used;
- The hair you are working with;
- The result you want to achieve.

Some products are designed to be applied directly from the bottle or tube, whilst others need to be mixed with hydrogen peroxide and other ingredients, and applied with a brush.

Always follow the manufacturers' instructions.

6.1 Application of temporary colorants

Mousses and gels

Mousses and gels should be applied to clean hair which should also have been towel-dried because excess moisture in the hair will dilute the product. Spread the product onto your hands and then distribute evenly through the hair. Comb through to ensure that the product is evenly distributed. Then style the hair.

Some gels – depending on the manufacturers' instructions – can also be applied when the hair is dry and the styling is complete. Use your fingers to place the gel exactly where you want it.

Setting lotions and rinses

These products should be applied to clean, towel-dried hair. Sprinkle the colour directly from the bottle or applicator onto the hair making sure that it is evenly distributed. Comb through the hair and then continue with styling.

Alternatively, you can apply this type of colour with a brush from a bowl, following the same pattern as you would for a regrowth tint application, and then comb the hair to distribute the colour onto the ends. This is a good method if you are trying to disguise a regrowth with a temporary colour.

Gels, sprays, paints and crayons

These should be applied when the hair is dry and styling is complete. Apply gels and paints exactly where you want them with your fingers or a small painting or make-up brush. Crayons are applied like lipstick to the hair. Coloured sprays are applied from a distance of 15–20 cm, and you may need to protect the areas you don't want to colour by using some type of screen, such as tissue or tin-foil.

6.2 Application of semi-permanent colorants

Semi-permanent colorants can either be applied to dry, unwashed hair, or to shampooed, towel-dried hair, so always check the manufacturers' instructions.

Semi-permanent colorants are usually applied to hair that has been shampooed and towel-dried. Shampooing will not only remove dirt and other debris from the hair but will also help to open the cuticle which enables the colorant to penetrate the hair shaft. Towel-drying hair after it has been shampooed will remove any excess moisture which could dilute the effect of the colorant.

Many semi-permanent colorants can be applied to the hair directly from the bottle or tube while others may need to be applied with either a tint brush or sponge, or from an applicator flask. Whichever application technique is used, it is important that you apply the colorant evenly so that the result is not patchy.

Application techniques:

- Applying directly from bottle, tube or applicator flask;
- Applying colour with a brush or sponge from a bowl.

You will only be able to apply the colorant directly from the tube or bottle if there is no need to mix two shades of the colorant together. You would not achieve satisfactory results if you attempted to mix the colours together once they were on the client's hair! If it is necessary to mix the colorant, you could use an applicator flask to measure amounts of the product you need and then, placing your finger over the opening of the nozzle, give it a shake to blend the colours together. Most manufacturers are aware that many hairdressers prefer to apply the colorant directly from the product container so they have nozzles on the bottles and tubes to make application easier.

The application begins at the nape where the hair is least receptive, and is evenly applied from the roots to the points. Gentle massage and combing with a wide-toothed comb will ensure the colorant is evenly distributed. The colour is then allowed to develop for the time recommended by the manufacturer.

The development time can be anything between 5 and 45 minutes depending on the type of product you are using. The instructions may suggest that the client's head is covered with a plastic cap during the development to help the colorant work more quickly. Some manufacturers may suggest you place the client under a hood dryer or other form of heat, which will assist the colour molecules to penetrate the hair shaft.

6.3 Application of quasi-permanent or cosmetic colorants

Quasi-permanent (or cosmetic) colorants can either be applied to freshly shampooed hair which has been towel-dried or to dry hair, so check the manufacturers' instructions. They are normally applied using an applicator bottle or flask or from a bowl using a tint brush.

These types of colorants are usually applied to the entire hair, straight through from roots to ends, but this is not always the case. Sometimes, the roots will need a longer colour development time than the ends. This application technique would be used in the following situations:

- It is a subsequent colour application and there is a definite demarcation line between the regrowth and the previously coloured hair. Failing to apply the colorant to the root area first might result in colour build-up on the lengths of the hair and a lack of coverage on the roots.
- The lengths and ends are particularly porous resulting in these parts of the hair requiring a shorter development time.

6.4 Application techniques of permanent oxidation colorants

Application

There are three main methods of application for tint which are:

- Regrowth application;
- Full head application (virgin hair);
- Partial colouring (lowlights, block colouring, etc.).

Tint is always applied to dry, unwashed hair except when it is applied as a toner after pre-lightening with a bleach, when it is applied to towel-dried hair. The reason for omitting the shampoo before applying a tint is that the body's natural oil (sebum) helps to protect the hair and scalp from the chemicals contained in tints. Also, the action of shampooing has a tendency to stimulate the scalp, bringing the blood to the surface of the skin, making the scalp more sensitive to the tint.

There might be the odd occasion when you will need to shampoo the hair before the hair is tinted but such instances will be rare. Pre-shampooing is only necessary when the hair is so heavily coated with oil or styling products (such as gel or pomade) that the tint would be unable to penetrate this barrier. A single application of shampoo, cool water and minimal massage is used if pre-shampooing is necessary. After shampooing, the hair will need drying before the tint is applied.

Whichever application technique you use, you should work in a neat, speedy and competent manner. Applying a tint for a regrowth application should not be a lengthy process and most salons would estimate that it should take no longer than 10–15 minutes for an average head of hair with a 1 cm regrowth.

Development

The tint is left to develop either naturally or with the additional heat provided by an infra-red appliance such as a Climazon (see Fig. 7.2). Using additional heat accelerates the development time, reducing it by as much as 50%. However, you will need to check the product instructions to see whether acceleration of the development time is recommended by the manufacturer. Do not cover the hair with a plastic cap because this can smudge the tint to areas other than those you wish to colour. If no additional heat is used, the normal development time for the roots will be about 20–30 minutes.

For a regrowth application, once the roots have developed, the hairdresser needs to check whether the tint should be combed through to the middle lengths and ends. This is only necessary when the previously tinted hair has faded and you need to restore the lost colour. The best way to determine if combing through is

necessary is to scrape off some tint from the roots using the back
of a comb, and compare the newly coloured regrowth with the
colour of the ends. If there is an obvious colour difference, the tint
will need to be taken through to the ends to achieve an even
colour result.

6.5   Tint – regrowth application technique

When tinting a regrowth you will be working on hair which has
been tinted before, and the client will want the newly grown hair
coloured to match the existing colour on the middle lengths and
ends. If the client is a regular visitor to your salon, there will be a
record card that will tell you which tint should be applied and the
length of the development time. This card should be referred to
and the client should be consulted to determine whether any
changes need to be made to the formula before the tint is mixed. If
the client is new to your salon, you will need to carry out an
analysis of the hair to determine which products will produce the
desired target colour.

*N.B. A tint should not be applied unless the client has been given
a skin test to determine whether they are allergic to the chemicals
contained in this type of colorant.*

Application techniques will vary between salons due to personal
preference, so I have chosen to describe one of the most commonly
used methods.

Method

1   Divide the hair into four main
    sections from the front hairline
    to the nape and from ear to ear
    across the crown as shown in
    Fig. 6.1. Each of the four sec-
    tions is then secured with clips.
2   Beginning at the nape, apply
    the tint to the regrowth area
    continuing up to the crown
    where the partings form a cross.

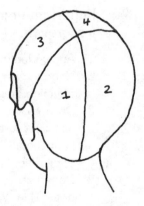

Fig. 6.1   Hair divided into four
main sections in preparation
for a regrowth tint application.

3 Start making narrow, horizontal partings at the nape area of one of the back sections, which are not deeper than 1 cm and apply the tint carefully to the regrowth. Continue taking these narrow sections, applying the tint as you progress up to the crown as shown in Fig. 6.2.

4 This procedure is repeated on the other back section.

5 The two front sections can then be treated, but instead of horizontal partings, the hair is parted so that the hair is always taken back from the face, so that the chances of the tint dripping or splashing into the client's eyes are reduced.

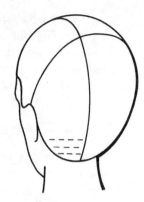

Fig. 6.2 Making 1 cm partings from the nape up to the crown to apply the tint to.

6 After applying the tint to the regrowth, your application needs to be cross-checked to ensure that no area has been missed. This is done by taking narrow partings in an *opposite* direction to the way you parted the hair to apply the tint. In other words, where you made horizontal partings for the hair at the back, it is cross-checked by taking vertical partings. Any area you notice that has been missed is covered with the tint during the cross-checking.

6.6 Important points to remember when tinting a regrowth.

1 Apply plenty of product.

2 Narrow (1 cm) partings ensure complete coverage of the regrowth area.

3 Do not overlap the tint onto the previously coloured hair as this will cause 'banding'. A darker line appears where this has happened.

4 Avoid dabbing on the tint – lay the product onto the hair.

5 Do not apply tint unnecessarily to the neck, ears or other parts of the skin. We are in the business of colouring hair not skin!

Before a tint is removed, the hairdresser should check that the result is even along the hair shaft. This check is made by doing a strand test which is fully explained in Chapter 2. Refer to Chapter 7 for an explanation of how tints are removed from the hair after development.

6.7 Tint – refreshing faded ends (combing through)

If tint is to be applied to previously coloured hair that has faded, the remaining tint in the bowl is usually diluted with equal parts of warm water. The addition of the water dilutes the strength of the hydrogen peroxide in the tint mixture so that it acts more as a semi-permanent colorant than a tint, restoring the lost colour. Depending on the degree of fade, the tint is left on the hair for 5 to 15 minutes before it is rinsed off.

6.8 Tint – virgin hair application technique

Virgin hair is hair that has not been treated with chemicals. This term is also used to describe hair that may have been given a perm or a semi-permanent colour, but has not been subjected to a process where colouring chemicals penetrate the hair shaft and alter the internal composition of the cortex.

It is a major decision for a client to opt for a complete and permanent colour change. Understandably, many clients will need reassurance from their hairdresser during the colouring procedure and need to feel confident about what is being done to their hair.

A first application takes longer to carry out than a regrowth application because the effect of body heat needs to be taken into account. Heat given off by the scalp speeds up the development of tints. The lengths and ends of hair do not receive this body heat because they are too far away from the heat source. Therefore, if the tint is applied through the entire length of the hair from roots to ends, the hair nearest the scalp will develop more quickly than the hair at the ends.

To enable hair to develop so that the end result is evenly coloured throughout its length, the tint is applied and partly developed on the middle lengths and ends *before* it is applied to the roots.

Method

1 Divide the hair into four main sections as you would for a regrowth application.

2 Beginning at the nape, make 1 cm horizontal partings and apply the tint to the middle lengths and ends of the hair to within 1 cm of the scalp.

3 When the tint has been applied to all the hair *except* the roots, leave the hair to develop for half the time recommended by the product manufacturer.

4 When this time is up, mix fresh tint and apply to the roots refreshing the tint that has already been applied to the lengths and ends.

5 Allow the hair to develop for the full development time.

6.9 Application of bleach

Bleach is applied in two ways:

(1) to a regrowth;
(2) to virgin hair.

Bleach – regrowth application technique

This service is carried out on hair that has been bleached before and the purpose of the client's visit is to match the newly grown hair (the regrowth) to the colour of the rest of the hair. Obviously, this is not as time-consuming as a virgin application.

Starting at the darkest part (usually the nape), apply the bleach to the regrowth, following the same pattern as you would for the applications described earlier. When you finish your application you should cross-check to ensure all the regrowth has been treated with the bleach.

6.10 Bleach – virgin hair application technique

1 Divide the hair into four main sections (forehead to nape and from ear to ear across the crown) and secure with clips.

Application (first stage)

2 Beginning at the base of one of the back sections, part off a horizontal mesh of hair that is no deeper than 1 cm and clip the remaining hair in the section out of your way. Lay the mesh of hair across the palm of your hand as shown in Fig. 6.3 and apply the bleach to within 2–3 cm of the scalp *only*. Place a narrow strip of cotton wool along the root area where there is

no bleach and part off your next
mesh. (The cotton wool stops any of
the bleach touching the roots at this
stage.)

3 Continue working up the head towards
the crown until that back section is
finished. Repeat on the other back
section.

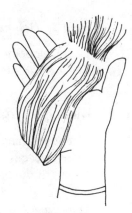

Fig. 6.3 Position for
applying bleach to
lengths and ends.

4 When the back is completed, begin parting your meshes on
one of the front sections. Work towards the front hairline and
take care to avoid any bleach dripping or splashing into the
client's eyes. Repeat this on the other side, completing the first
stage of this application at the front hairline.

Development

5 Allow the bleach to develop until you can see that *half* the
degree of lift required has been achieved. This means visually
checking the hair by performing a strand test. If the target
colour is six shades lighter than the client's natural base colour,
allow the hair to lighten only three shades before you move
onto the second stage of the application.

Application (second stage)

6 Mix *fresh* bleach of the same strength and remove the cotton
wool strips that were used to keep the bleach away from the
roots. Apply the bleach to the root area following the same
pattern you used for the initial application (i.e. starting at the
nape). As you apply the bleach to the roots, also refresh that
already on the middle lengths and ends by applying new
bleach. You need to do this to ensure that the bleach on the
middle lengths and ends has the necessary lightening power.
Cross-check your application to ensure that all the hair is
treated with the bleach.

Final development

7   Develop the bleach until the hair has lightened sufficiently. Check this by visually testing hair on several areas of the head.

6.11   Bleach – virgin hair application (longer than 20 cm)

When bleaching hair which is longer than 20 cm for the first time a different sequence has to be followed to ensure an even colour result. This is because the differing degrees of porosity along the hair's length will affect how quickly the bleach will lighten the hair. The longer (and subsequently older) the hair is, the more porous it will be because it has been subject to more wear and tear.

The ends of the hair are the most porous (because they are the oldest) and will therefore be more receptive to bleach than the less porous areas. Porous hair has a damaged cuticle which allows chemicals to penetrate the hair shaft more easily than hair with a closed cuticle. Although the root area will not be as porous because it is the newest hair, remember that the warmth of the head will mean the roots will lighten more quickly than the ends. The middle lengths of the hair will be most resistant to bleaching so this area will require a longer development time and hence this is where application starts. The order for bleach application on this length of hair is shown in Fig. 6.4.

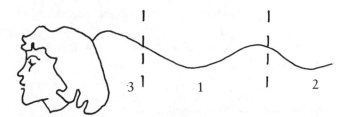

Fig. 6.4   Differing degrees of porosity along hair's length.

Application (first stage)

1   Prepare your client and mix the bleach according to the manufacturer's instructions.
2   Divide the hair into four main sections (forehead to nape and from ear to ear across the crown) and secure with clips.
3   Starting at the base of one of the back sections, horizontally part off a mesh of hair that is no deeper than 1 cm and clip

the remaining hair out of your way. Lay the mesh across the palm of your hand as shown in Fig. 6.3 and apply the bleach to within 2–3 cm of the scalp only. Place a narrow strip of cotton wool along the root area where there is no bleach and part off your next mesh. (The cotton wool strip prevents the bleach from coming into contact with the root area at this stage.)

4   Continue working up the head towards the crown until all of that back section is completed. Repeat this on the other back section.

5   When the back is complete, begin parting your meshes on one of the front sections. Work towards the front hairline and take care to avoid any dripping or splashing of the bleach product. Repeat this on the other side.

6   Allow the bleach to develop until you can see that half the degree of lift required has been achieved. This means visually checking the hair by performing a strand test. For example, if the target colour is six shades lighter than the client's natural hair colour, allow the hair to lighten by three shades only.

Application (second stage)

7   Apply the bleach to the points of the hair then mix *fresh bleach* of the same strength for the roots.

8   Remove the cotton wool strips that were placed at the roots and apply the bleach to the root area and apply some of this fresh bleach mixture to the middle lengths.

9   Cross-check your work to ensure no areas have been missed.

10   Allow the hair to lighten and when it has reached the desired degree of lightness, rinse the bleach from the hair using tepid water and then gently shampoo.

11   You may want to apply a pastel toner in the form of a semi-quasi-permanent or permanent colorant to achieve the target colour.

6.12   Case study: Bleaching long, virgin hair

Remember that this example is only a guide, and that the application and products you use depend on the hair you are working with and your skill.

Target colour – pale ash blonde – base 10.
Natural base – base 5 with slight warmth.

Condition – slightly porous on ends. (Hair is approximately 25 cm long.)
Previous colouring – none.
Products – bleach, followed by a toner.
Application – virgin application.

1 Pre-lightener was mixed.
2 Pre-lightener was applied to the middle lengths only and developed until half the degree of lift was achieved. (This took approximately 20 minutes to develop.)
3 Fresh pre-lightener (of the same strength) was mixed and applied to the root area.
4 The pre-lightener was then applied to the ends. To refresh the middle lengths, more of the product was applied over the top of the pre-lightener already applied.
5 The hair was then developed until it reached a very pale yellow. (This took approximately 45 minutes.)
6 The pre-lightener was rinsed from the hair which was then shampooed and conditioned (with a non-barrier forming conditioner).
7 The hair was towel-dried and the toner was mixed. 10/01 and 20 vol hydrogen peroxide was applied straight through from roots to ends, and developed for 20–25 minutes.
8 The hair was then shampooed and given a conditioning treatment.

In all, the colouring alone took about two hours to complete.

6.13 Highlighting and lowlighting

What is highlighting?

Highlighting is a technique for lightening selected strands of hair using any of the following methods:

- Cap or plastic bag
- Foil
- Easi-Meche
- Cling film.

What is lowlighting?

The lowlighting technique darkens selected strands of hair using the same methods as for highlighting – but creating the opposite effect.

6.14 The cap or plastic bag method of highlighting or lowlighting

1   Comb hair into finished style.
2   Position the cap or plastic bag over the head, ensuring that the fit is as snug as possible. (See Figs. 6.5 and 6.6.)
3   Using a crochet hook, pull through the strands of hair to be coloured.
4   Comb strands with a fine-toothed comb.
5   Apply your chosen tint or pre-lightener. Cover the head with another plastic bag or foil to speed the development.
6   After development, remove any bag or foil used to speed the development. At this stage, do *not* remove the cap or plastic bag through which the strands have been pulled. Rinse the colorant from the strands. (If you are *not* going to apply a toner, proceed to point 7. If you *do* intend to use a toner, skip next point and proceed to 8.)
7   Apply a little conditioner to the strands. *Gently* pull off the cap or plastic bag. Shampoo and condition hair.
8   Give the strands one gentle shampoo and towel-dry.
9   Apply the toner to the strands and allow to develop.
10 Rinse toner from strands. Apply a little conditioner.
11 *Gently* pull off cap or bag. Shampoo and condition hair.

6.15 The foil method of highlighting or lowlighting

1   Prepare strips of foil, the same length as the hair you are working on but no wider than 10 cm. Try to keep the foil as smooth as possible – crumpled foil is hard to work with. Lay the foil *shiny side down*, and make a fold at one end, as in Fig. 6.7. This gives you a less flimsy, straight edge to work with.
2   Divide hair into 9 sections (Fig. 6.8). You will carry out this procedure from sections 1–9. Zig-zag out 0.5 cm of hair around entire hair line and on either side of the parting. When the lights grow out, a regrowth will be less noticeable if this is done.

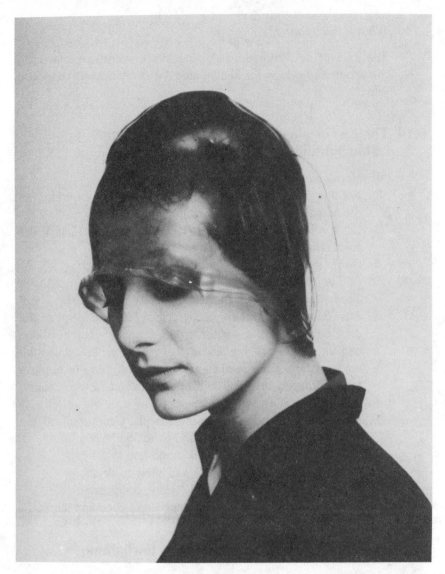

Fig. 6.5 Cap method highlights. (Reproduced courtesy of L'Oréal.)

3 Prepare the product(s) you will be using to colour the hair. If using more than one colour, it is a good idea to label the bowls, as many tints look the same once mixed.

4 Working from the base of section 1, weave out the strands of hair to be coloured. Make sure that these strands are equal in size and evenly spaced.

5 Lay a strip of foil underneath the strands, dull-side uppermost, with the folded edge *as close as possible* to the scalp.

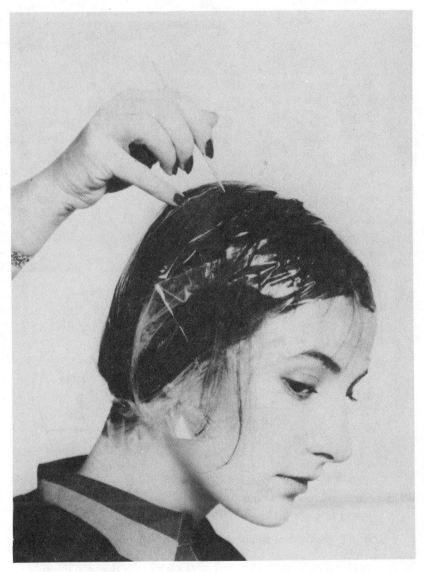

Fig. 6.6 Plastic bag method highlights. (Reproduced courtesy of L'Oréal.)

Hold the foil firmly in place, with your thumb and forefinger.

6 Using your other hand, apply your product to the strands using a tint brush (Fig. 6.9). Make sure you apply the product to within 0.5 cm of the folded edge *only*. Leaving this gap allows for the natural expansion of the colouring product.

7 Fold the strip of foil in half so that the two edges meet (Fig. 6.10).

Dull side

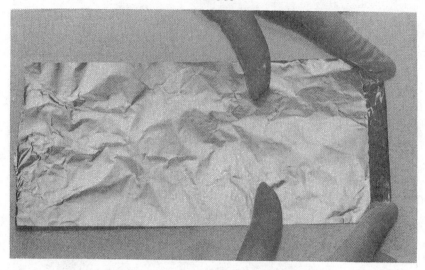

Folded side

Fig. 6.7 Preparation of foil for highlighting.

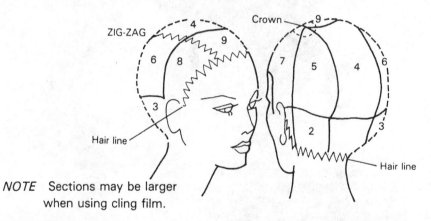

NOTE Sections may be larger when using cling film.

Fig. 6.8 Method of sectioning the hair for foil. (Reproduced courtesy of L'Oréal.)

8 Now fold the two outside *edges* toward the centre to make a packet (Fig. 6.11).

9 To help prevent the product from seeping out of the foil packet, you can do *either* of the following:

- Wrap a small strip of cotton wool around the root area of the packet and secure with a clip, *or*
- Wrap a narrow strip of folded foil around the root area of the packet and secure with a clip, *or*

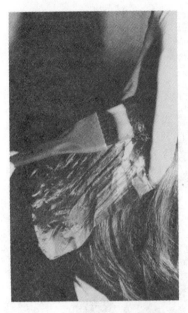

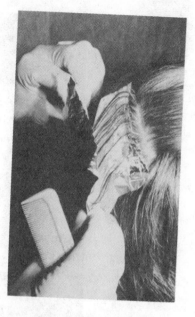

Fig. 6.9 Applying product to woven strands.

Fig. 6.10 Folding foil.

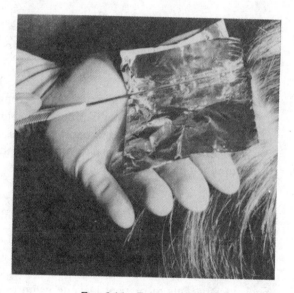

Fig. 6.11 Folding foil.

- Place the pointed end of your tail-comb across the root area of the packet and hold firmly. Lift the packet up so that a deep crease is achieved where you held your comb. This crease will act as a 'seal' (Fig. 6.12).

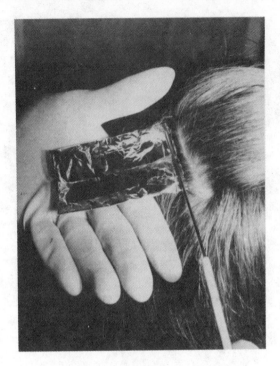

Fig. 6.12 Sealing foil.

10 Take your next mesh of hair, approximately 1 cm above the foil packet, and repeat the weaving technique. Continue working through sections of hair, finishing with number 9. As you will be working from the nape upwards, the foil packets will lie on top of each other with the hair that is not being coloured lying in between (Fig. 6.13).

Important points for foil colouring (highlighting and lowlighting)

- Do not apply too much product because it will expand and could seep out of the packet.
- Seal your packets to prevent leakage using one of the techniques listed.
- Ensure that your weaving is equally spaced and that the strands are the same thickness.
- If using pre-lightener, remember to check development *regularly*. This is done by opening the foil packets. If the hair is light enough, simply rinse at a back-basin, or wipe the product

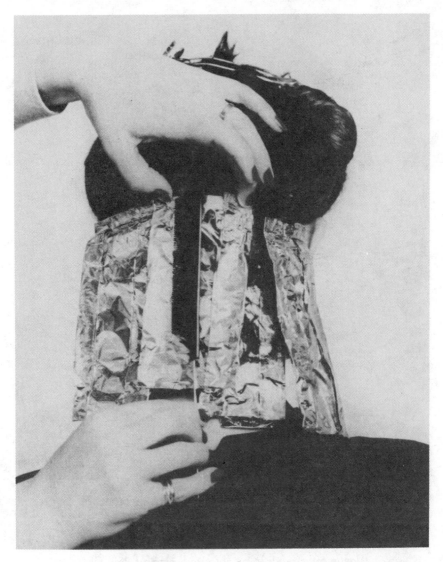

Fig. 6.13 Foil method highlights. (Reproduced by courtesy of L'Oréal.)

from the hair using wet cotton wool. If it is not ready, close and reseal the packet and continue development.

6.16 The cling-film method of highlighting or lowlighting

1 The cling-film method (Fig. 6.14) is similar to both foil and Easi-Meche methods [6.17] but there is no need to section hair into nine parts as larger areas of hair can be treated at one time. Always begin at the nape, working upwards.

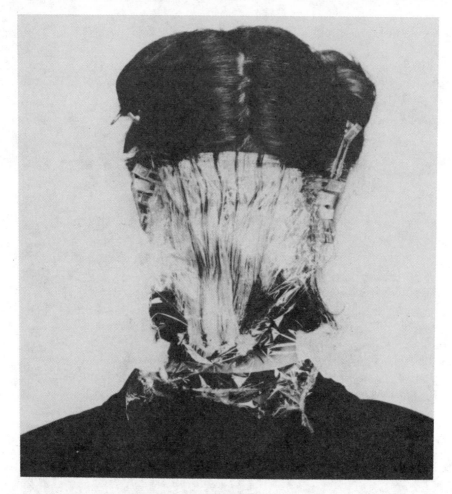

Fig. 6.14 Cling-film method of highlighting. (Reproduced courtesy of L'Oréal.)

2 Weave out strands to be coloured, placing cling film underneath the strands. Lay the meshes onto a spatula and apply product.
3 Place another sheet of cling film over the strands and seal it to the cling film that the strands are resting on. Remove the spatula.
4 Continue working through the sections of hair.
5 Develop the colour as normal.

6.17 The Easi-Meche method of highlighting or lowlighting

1 Prepare the hair as for the foil technique.

2   Weave out the strands to be coloured. Peel back the clear sheet of the Easi-Meche. Place the white sheet underneath, as close as possible to the roots. Stick the strands to the blue adhesive strip. (You now have two hands free to work with.)

3   Paint on the product to just above the dark blue adhesive strip. Place the edge of the clear sheet slightly above the lighter blue line. Seal in a downwards movement at the edges only (Fig. 6.15).

4   Continue working through the sections of hair, finishing with number 9.

Special advantages of Easi-Meche

- Leaves two hands free to work with.
- No need to unwrap packets to check development.
- They are ready to use (they come in three lengths, and can be cut to half the original width).
- Self-sealing.
- Comfortable for client.
- For extra-long hair, Easi-Meche can be joined together with the adhesive strips to produce any length of package.

6.18 Henna – application technique

The consistency of henna can make it difficult to apply. You are advised to use a tint brush to apply it to the hair. Please note that henna stains the skin and that you should not apply the mixture to the client's scalp. The henna mixture should be applied to the root area of the hair as close as possible to the scalp without actually coming into contact with the skin.

Henna is applied straight through from roots to points, covering the whole length of the hair using the same application pattern as described earlier [6.5]. The only time this is not done is when there is an obvious regrowth, and colouring the middle lengths and ends again, would result in an uneven colour.

6.19 Camomile – application technique

If applying a camomile paste, the mixture is applied in the same manner as described above for henna. If you are applying the camomile as a rinse, the solution is poured through the hair (at the back-basin) as a final rinse. An applicator bottle should be used to ensure the solution can be evenly distributed through the hair.

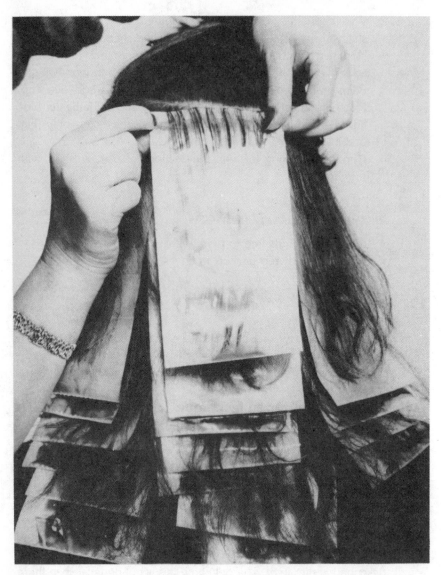

Fig. 6.15   Easi-Meche method of highlighting. (Reproduced courtesy of L'Oréal.)

6.20   Colour application – at a glance

The methods of colorant application are shown in Fig. 6.16.

6.21   Revision questions

1   How often will a client need to have their roots tinted to maintain the colour?

	Brush	Sponge	Applicator flask/bottle	Direct from tube/bottle
Temporary	√		√	√
Semi-permanent	√	√	√	√
Quasi-permanent	√		√	
Permanent tint	√		√	
Bleach	√		√	
Henna	√			
Camomile*	√		√	

√ = suitable application technique

* = brush for camomile paste, applicator flask for camomile solution

Fig. 6.16 Methods of application.

2 How would you apply a temporary colour contained in a setting lotion?

3 What is the purpose of *combing through* a tint?

4 Why should a regrowth tint application not overlap onto previously coloured hair?

5 How is hair prepared for application of a semi-permanent colorant?

6 What can be added to henna paste to improve the hair's shine or intensify colour results?

7 What are the two methods of preparing camomile?

8 How is a quasi-permanent (or cosmetic) colorant prepared?

9 Where should you start a regrowth bleach application?

10 When applying cap highlights why should bleach not be mixed before all the strands have been pulled through the cap?

11 How is foil prepared for weave (foil) highlights?

12 Why is it recommended that henna is not applied directly to the scalp?

13 What is the difference between highlights and lowlights?

14 When doing a first time bleach application why is it necessary to apply bleach to the lengths and ends of the hair before the roots?

15   What might happen if bleach was applied to previously bleached hair?

16   Why is conditioner applied to highlighted strands before removing the highlighting cap?

17   Will a hot salon make bleach work more quickly or more slowly?

18   List five important points to be remembered when applying tint to a regrowth.

19   List four methods which could be used for highlighting hair.

6.22 Advanced questions

1   Describe how you would carry out a first time bleach application to hair which is longer than 20 cm.

2   Describe the various techniques used when dealing with tinted hair that has faded ends, explaining when each would be used.

3   Describe how you would carry out a set of weave highlights on hair that was over 20 cm in length.

4   When doing cap highlights which are to be subsequently treated with a toner, describe the procedure for rinsing off the bleach.

Development and
Removal of Hair Colour

Development of hair colour

As with all products used in the salon, *always* read the manufacturers' instructions first.

7.1 Temporary colorants

This type of product has an instant colouring action, therefore no development time is required. Once the temporary colour is applied, you will be able to continue with styling. Some temporary colours are applied onto hair when styling is completed, while others are applied to damp hair.

7.2 Semi-permanent colorants

The development times of semi-permanent colours will vary according to the manufacturers who make them. *Usually*, these colorants require a development time of between 5 and 30 minutes. The longer the colorant is allowed to develop, the more obvious the final colour result. Porous hair, which will be receptive to the product because of the open cuticle, may require a shorter development time than hair in good condition. The client can have the colour applied at the backwash or styling position and can be left there while the colour takes. Make sure that none of the product drips or runs onto the client's clothing or face. If this seems likely due to the consistency of the product you are using, cover the hair with a plastic bag.

Some semi-permanent colours require heat to develop properly, in which case either a hood drier or an infra-red accelerator is used. If a hood drier is used (Fig. 7.1) ensure that the product will not run onto the face or clothing by covering the hair with a plastic bag and securing it with a hairnet or clip. The ears can be protected with small pads of cotton wool. Always switch on the hood drier several minutes before using, so that it is at a comfortable tempera-

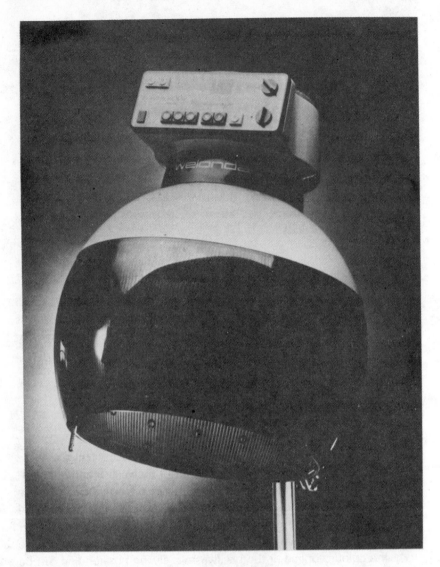

Fig. 7.1 An example of a modern hood drier. The Futura 2002 Electronic Superstar (by Wella).

ture for the client. Do make it obvious to the client that you will be timing the development of the colour and how long he or she will be expected to stay under the drier. Many clients feel forgotten if they are not told and may begin to panic!

Infra-red accelerators will also supply the necessary heat to develop hair colours. The infra-red heat can be supplied from a Solar or from a Climazon (Fig. 7.2). Both of these produce heat which does not disturb the hair, unlike the warm air flow from a

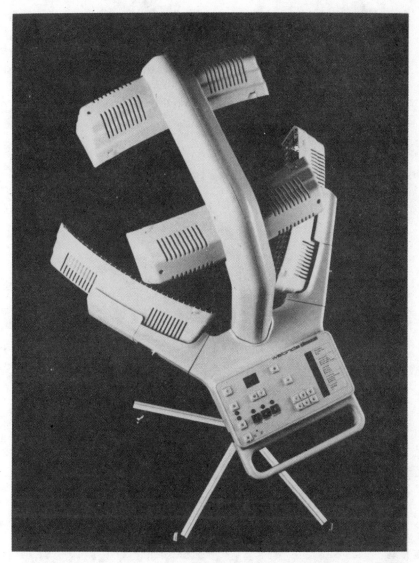

Fig. 7.2 Wellonda Climazon (by Wella).

hair drier. For this reason, plastic caps to cover the hair are not necessary, although long hair may need to be clipped-up at the back to ensure that it receives the heat from the appliance. As infra-red light can be dangerous to the eyes, position the appliance so that any light given off from the bulbs is directed at the client's hair. Both Solars and Climazons have timers incorporated into the control panel, so the development time is set, and the machine will automatically switch itself off when that time has passed.

Steamers are *not* recommended by most manufacturers to develop hair colours. Steamers (see Fig. 7.3) work on the basis of heating water, contained in a special reservoir, and converting it into steam. This moist heat travels up to the hood of the appliance where the client's head would be. Obviously, any moisture will dilute the colour on the hair, making the results less effective.

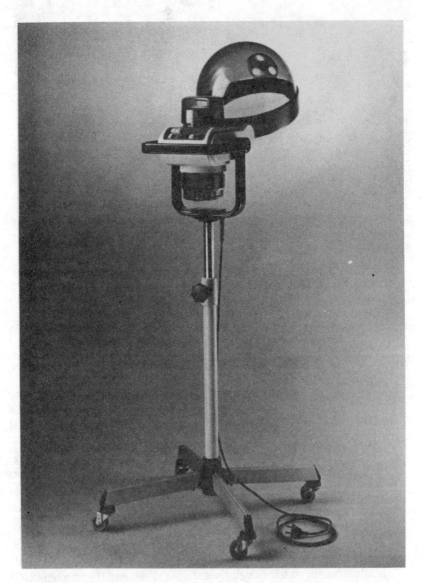

Fig. 7.3 Wellapor P5 Steamer (by Wella).

7.3   Quasi-permanent or cosmetic colorants

These types of colorants require a development time of between 5 and 20 minutes, depending on the type of hair you are working with and whether or not you use an external source of heat (such as infra-red lamps) to speed the development time. If you are applying the colorant to a regrowth, the root area may require some development time before the colorant is taken through to the lengths and ends of the hair. Check the manufacturers' instructions.

7.4   Permanent oxidation colorants

Development times of permanent colorants vary from product to product so it is important to read the manufacturers' instructions. On average, the time is 25–45 minutes, but will vary according to the product you are using and the type of hair you are working with. It is important that you allow the tint to develop for the maximum time on the regrowth (virgin hair) but you may want to comb the tint through the lengths and ends for the last five minutes or so to level out the colour of the faded areas.

Infra-red accelerators can be used to speed up the development. Plastic bags, towels or tin-foil should not be used to cover the hair during development as these might disturb the product and your careful application. When infra-red accelerators are used to develop tints, the process is much quicker. For example, if 30 minutes was needed to develop the regrowth, only 15 minutes would be necessary if using a Solar or Climazon appliance. However, some manufacturers advise against the use of external heat for developing tints, as they believe this causes more colour fading.

7.5   Bleach

A bleach is left on the hair until the desired degree of lightness is achieved. Therefore, bleaches are developed by observing the lightening process at regular intervals. On average, bleaches are left on the hair for 15–60 minutes, but this depends upon the strength of the product being used and the hair type you are working with. Hair containing warm colours (that is, natural gold or copper glints) will take longer to lighten than hair without warm colours. This is because pheomelanin (the red and yellow pigment in hair) is more difficult to eliminate as the colour molecules are small and scattered in the cortex. The use of external heat (infra-red, driers, steamers, etc.) is *not* advised. Heat may cause severe damage to the skin and hair and you will have less control over the lightening process. It is worth noting that it is kinder to the hair to have a milder bleach on it for a longer development time than a strong bleach for a shorter time. Damage to the hair *will* occur if, for example, 60 vol hydrogen peroxide is mixed with powder bleach and applied to cap highlights, especially if a steamer or other source of heat is used to speed the lightening of the hair. It is useful to note that when the salon is warmer, bleaches will work more quickly, so check development at regular intervals.

7.6 Henna

The development time for henna varies according to the result required. The longer the henna is allowed to stay on the hair, the more obvious the change of hair colour will be. *Usually*, it takes 30–60 minutes to develop *with heat*. However, it can take up to two hours! As the best results are normally obtained when the henna has been baked until it is hard, a hood drier is the ideal source of heat. Wrap the hair in tin-foil (clipping the hair up if it is long) and hold the foil in place with a hairnet, clips or tape. As the client is likely to be under the hood drier for a long time, do make sure he or she has plenty to read, is comfortable, and is supplied with refreshments. As henna stains skin as well as hair, do clean any marks off the hairline, neck or ears *before* placing the client under the hood drier.

7.7 Camomile

If a camomile paste has been applied, it will need to be developed in the same way as henna. The longer the camomile paste is left on the hair, the stronger the yellow cast will be on the hair. If the camomile is applied as a final rinse, there is no development time.

Removal (rinsing) of hair colours

7.8 Temporary colorants

Temporary colorants are *not* rinsed or shampooed after the application. They have an instant colouring action that lasts until the next shampoo. Any accidental stains on the face, neck or ears should be removed with a swab of damp cotton wool immediately after the application.

7.9 Semi-permanent colorants

To remove a semi-permanent colour, add a little warm water to the hair and gently massage the scalp and hair. This helps to loosen the colour and helps prevent staining of the scalp. After the massage, give the hair a long, warm rinse. Do this until the water runs clear. There is no need to use shampoo, and as many semi-permanents contain built-in conditioners, the use of conditioning cream is not usually required. Some products may have their own special conditioner included in the package. These are often not rinsed from the hair, so check the instructions. Once the colour is completely rinsed from the hair it can be styled. When dry, the hair will be silky, shiny and glowing with colour.

7.10 Quasi-permanent or cosmetic colorants

Add a little warm water to the hair and massage to gently loosen the colorant from the hair. Rinse the hair thoroughly until the water runs clear. There is no need to shampoo the hair if it was shampooed before the colorant was applied.

7.11 Permanent oxidation colorants

Permanent colorants must be removed properly to avoid leaving stains on the client's skin. Tint will come away from the hair and scalp very easily if it is *emulsified*. To emulsify, add a little water to the hair and massage the whole scalp. The massage loosens the tint from the hair and scalp. Gradually, as you add more water and continue with your massage, the tint will begin to take on the appearance of a shampoo and may even begin to foam. Now thoroughly rinse the colour from the hair. Give the hair one shampoo with either a cream or pH-balanced shampoo. A pH-balanced shampoo will help the hair return to its normal pH level, close the cuticle and help neutralize any traces of the tint left on the hair. As tints have a pH of between 9.5 and 10.5 the hair will benefit from this type of shampoo because they are slightly acid, having a pH level of about 5.

Always condition the hair after a tint application as the alkaline level of these products has a drying effect on the hair, even though many contain conditioning agents. When the hair is styled, make sure that your client is positioned in the best possible light to see the new colour. If necessary, take them to the window so that it can be seen in natural daylight.

Recommend to your client that he or she uses a pH-balanced shampoo or conditioner at home, as these help close the cuticle, thereby helping to prevent colour fade.

7.12 Bleach

Bleach has a tendency to make the scalp sensitive, so long, *cool* rinsing will help reduce irritation. *Thoroughly* rinse all of the bleach from the hair then give one *gentle* shampoo using a pH-balanced product. *Always* condition the hair after applying a bleach as the pH level of bleaches (8.5–9.5) will tend to dry the hair.

N.B. If a permanent tint is to be applied as a toner after the bleach application, use a conditioner that will not form a barrier on the hair shaft, as this would prevent the tint from entering the hair.

7.13 Henna

Henna requires *very* long rinsing because the henna will have a 'crust' due to the hair being baked under a hood drier. Give a gentle shampoo to remove the small particles of colour from the hair and scalp. The scalp and hair will feel gritty if the henna is not removed thoroughly. After shampooing a conditioner can be applied, but because henna gives hair such a good shine, it is not normally needed. The hair can now be styled. When styling is complete, the hair will glow with colour and have an exceptional shine. Recommend that your client uses a henna shampoo at home as these contain small quantities of henna that will maintain and enhance the colour between applications.

7.14 Camomile

When removing a camomile paste from the hair you will need to rinse the hair thoroughly to remove all the colorant. After rinsing, the hair is shampooed and is ready for styling.

7.15 Revision questions

1 Which two colorants do not require a development time?
2 How does the use of an external source of heat (such as infra-red lamps) affect the development time of colorants?
3 What does the term *emulsify* mean when removing a colorant?
4 Why should cool water be used for rinsing off a bleach?

5 How are semi-permanent colorants removed from the hair?

6 If hair is very porous, would the development time for a semi-permanent be longer or shorter than that for hair in good condition?

7 How are henna and camomile pastes removed from the hair?

8 List at least two sources of external heat which may be used to speed the development time of colorants.

9 What are the benefits of using pH-balanced shampoos and conditioners after colour applications?

10 What type of conditioner should be applied to a freshly bleached head of hair before a toner is applied?

7.16 Advanced questions

1 Describe the effect of heat on the development time of colorants and state which types you would choose (and why) for the following:

(1) Henna
(2) Permanent oxidation tint
(3) Quasi-permanent or cosmetic colorant.

2 Explain how the use of pH-balanced shampoos and conditioners is beneficial to hair following colour treatment.

3 Describe the procedures taken to ensure that a client is not left with colorant stains on their skin after a colouring treatment.

4 Explain why the development of bleach has to be monitored in order to achieve the desired degree of lightness.

8

Colour Correction

There are only three corrections you can make to hair colour. These are:

(1)   Changing the tone;
(2)   Lightening;
(3)   Darkening.

It might not always be a dramatic change, but sometimes the colourist will need to carry out all three corrections on the same head!

You will need to spend time with your client discussing what the new colour is to be. If the client makes an impossible demand (e.g. light ash blonde on hair that has been tinted black for many years) the target colour must be renegotiated. The most limiting factor will be the hair itself. It may not be strong enough to take the colour correction needed to achieve the chosen colour. Other restrictions such as time, economics or personal whim must also be considered.

Colour correction is deciding:

• The problem that you are faced with;
• The new target colour;
• If necessary, how to achieve that colour on the regrowth;
• How to achieve that colour on the already coloured hair.

With this in mind I have selected several case studies of problems a colourist may face in the salon. I have chosen examples of the following:

• Colour stripping
• Re-colouring colour-stripped hair
• Dealing with faded middle lengths and ends
• Tinting pre-lightened hair darker
• Subduing unwanted tones in hair
• Lightening already pre-lightened hair
• Correcting highlights and lowlights.

8.1   Analysis for colour correction

Analysis for colour correction involves a sequenced assessment and identification of the present hair colour, the new target colour, the condition of the hair, and what process(es) will be necessary to achieve the result. Below is a helpful table, taking you through this complex sequence of analysis, stating the questions you should be asking yourself when carrying out this type of work.

What is the target colour?

What is the depth and tone of the regrowth?
Your choices are:
(a)   Tint regrowth
(b)   Pre-lighten regrowth
(c)   Leave natural colour.

Is there any white hair?
(See pre-softening [5.8] and colour analysis [4.3])

How damaged is the hair?
You will need to do the following tests:
(a)   Porosity
(b)   Elasticity.

What has been used on the hair?
You will need to:
(a)   Question your client (remember they will not always be totally truthful!);
(b)   Do an incompatibility test if you suspect a metallic colorant has been used;
(c)   Do a test cutting if in doubt of the result.

What is the problem?

Problem		Solution
Problem		*Solution*
Hair too light	→	Restore colour
Hair too dark	→	Remove colour
Wrong tone	→	Neutralize colour or clean-out

8.2   Colour stripping (reduction method)

What is it?

Colour stripping is the removal of the previous tint or the lightening of over-dark shades. The large coloured molecules are reduced in size until they are small enough to pass through the cuticle, where they are washed from the hair (see Fig. 8.1). Sometimes the colour does not strip out evenly because tints are a mixture of red, yellow and black molecules, and the red molecules may be left behind. Strippers can be either reducing agents (sulphites) or bleaches. As they must be alkaline (to open the cuticle to allow escape of colour) they will damage the hair.

Weak mixtures of colour stripper can be used to remove mild forms of colour build-up, or 'grabbing', from temporary or semi-permanent colours. In these cases, the product is usually mixed with a low strength hydrogen peroxide such as 10 vol (3%), or even water. However, as products vary, always read the manufacturers' instructions first.

Colour strippers are used mostly to remove dark colour from hair. It is *impossible* to achieve a lighter shade on previously tinted hair, by applying a lighter shade of tint. Too often, hairdressers

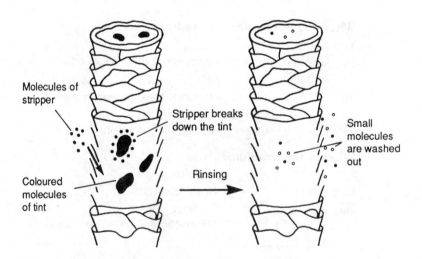

Colour can be stripped from the hair by using a reducing agent such as sodium bisulphite. This does the opposite to tinting, breaking up the large tint molecules so they can be washed from the hair.

Fig. 8.1   Stripping of colour by reduction.

think this is the case, and the result is darker than when they began! Just like painting a wall, the more coats of paint used, the deeper the colour. Unwanted dark hair colours *must* be removed first to avoid this.

Stripping colour from hair is really a job for experienced colourists only. A fast and even application is required, and the product strength is crucial to the result. Due to hair's uneven porosity, colour will be removed more easily from some areas (the more porous) than others. The colourist's application will therefore need to be selective, applying the stripper to the darker and more resistant areas first.

The regrowth is *not* treated with a colour stripper, so cotton wool strips are used to keep the product off the regrowth. The degree of colour removal will depend upon the amount to be stripped and it may be necessary to carry out a second application on the more stubborn areas.

The hair will take on various shades of red, orange and yellow after stripping a colour. Do not be alarmed as this is quite normal, but do remember to warn your client! He or she may be under the impression that this is the final result! Obviously, the next step is to achieve your target colour over the base the colour stripper has left you. As this 'undercoat' will not usually be 100% even, thought must be given to the application and the product you will be using to achieve the target shade.

The strength of colour stripper mixture will depend upon:

- The strength and intensity of the previous colour being used;
- The condition of the hair (the more damaged the hair is, the weaker the mixture should be).

See *Case Study (1): Colour stripping* [8.5].

8.3 Colour stripping using bleach

Bleach can be used to remove synthetic colorants from the hair but because they work differently to colour reducers, (bleaching is an oxidation process) the removal of unwanted colour may be slower and less effective. When using bleach as a colour stripper, you should take the same precautions as you would when working with a reducing colour stripper.

8.4 Cleaning-out/bleach bath

'Cleaning-out' is similar to colour stripping but the product used is a weak bleach mixture. You can use the cleaning-out technique if the colour you wish to get rid of is not dark and intense.

The cleaning-out technique is similar to colour-stripping, but is suitable only for getting rid of mild colour build-up or toners on bleached hair.

When to use the cleaning-out technique

Cleaning-out can be used:

(1) To remove a build-up temporary of semi-permanent colours;
(2) To clean out toners from bleached hair.

Basic procedure

1 Mix bleach bath, e.g. one part each of the following:
     3% (20 vol) hydrogen peroxide
     powder/paste bleach
     shampoo
     water
2 Apply to parts affected by the colour you want to remove.
3 Develop until colour is removed. (This could be as fast as five minutes on porous hair.)
4 Rinse and give one gentle shampoo.
5 Proceed with further colouring or styling.

8.5 Case Study (1): Colour stripping

Remember that this example should be regarded as a guide only and that the application and products you use depend on the hair you are working on and your skill.

- Target colour – light ash blonde.
- Natural base – dark blonde.
- Condition of hair – good.
- Previous colouring – chestnut brown tint.
- Problems – present colour too dark and too warm.
- Solution – strip colour on middle lengths and ends.

Basic procedure

1 Do not shampoo hair.
2 Mix colour stripper (accordng to manufacturer's instructions) and apply to the darkest parts of the hair first, *avoiding any regrowth*. Place strips of cotton wool between each section to prevent the stripper from seeping onto regrowth.
3 Observe the stripper lifting the colour. Do not leave your client as the colour may lighten suddenly.
4 Allow the stripper to lift the colour the desired degree (in this case three shades) and then rinse from the hair using cool water. Give one gentle shampoo and then towel-dry thoroughly.
5 At this stage of the process, you may find a second application necessary, or you will be able to determine what products you now need to use to achieve the target colour.
6 Always advise the client how to follow a home-care programme after such colouring.

8.6 Re-colouring colour-stripped hair

After stripping a colour, it is unlikely that you will end up with an even base colour on which to work. This is because the intensity of colour may have varied, and so lifted more easily in some places than others. It is also due to porosity, allowing the stripper to work more quickly on the more damaged parts of the hair. Your application should, of course, have taken these factors into consideration.

Colour analysis for the regrowth area will be as normal. Your choices are:

(1) Tinting the regrowth; or
(2) Pre-lightening the regrowth; or
(3) Leaving the natural colour.

For hair that has been stripped you must consider:

• The evenness of the base you are working on;
• The condition of the hair;
• The degree of warm tones left in the hair.

Problem	Solution
Uneven colour base	Consider stripping darker areas again to even out the base.
Excess warmth	Depending on your target colour you can either:
	(1) Pre-lighten areas to eliminate warmth; or
	(2) Choose a tint that will neutralize excess warmth.
Damaged hair	Remember that porous hair absorbs warmth so compensate by using warmer toned colours to prevent the results from looking flat.

See *Case Study (2): Re-colouring colour-stripped hair* [8.7].

8.7   Case Study (2): Re-colouring colour-stripped hair

Remember that this example is only a guide and that the application and products you use depend on the hair you are working on and your skill.

- Target colour – light ash blonde.
- Natural base – dark blonde.
- Condition of hair after stripping – ends now more porous.
- Base after stripping – yellow/orange.
- Problem – base too warm to achieve target colour.
- Solution – pre-lighten middle lengths and ends to remove unwanted warm tones.

Basic procedure

1 Dry hair completely. Mix bleach (according to manufacturer's instructions).
2 Apply bleach only to areas with excess warmth using strips of cotton wool between sections to prevent bleach from seeping onto regrowth.
3 Allow bleach to lighten, and eliminate unwanted yellow/orange tones.
4 Rinse bleach from hair using cool water and give one gentle shampoo. Dry hair completely. You should now be left with a less warm base for you to work on.

8.8 Dealing with faded middle lengths and ends

In the notes on colour application, it was explained how to refresh tinted hair that has faded. If the colour has faded more than usual (perhaps the client had a recent perm or returned from a holiday) a different procedure is followed.

A mistake hairdressers often make when trying to put colour back into faded hair is failing to add enough warmth to the hair. This results in a flat colour which will not hold. Porous hair absorbs warmth so you must compensate for this by using a warmer colour.

N.B. If the colour fade is extreme, or if the client wishes to change to a darker or redder shade, pre-pigmentation may be necessary (see [8.10]).

See Case Study (3): Dealing with faded middle lengths and ends [8.9].

8.9 Case Study (3): Dealing with faded middle lengths and ends

Remember that this example is only a guide and that the application and products you use depend on the hair you are working on and your skill.

- Target colour – 9/03.
- Natural base – 7/0.
- Colour previously used – 9/03 + 30 vol (9%) peroxide.
- Condition of hair – middle lengths and ends porous due to harsh physical abuse (e.g. regular use of tongs).
- Problem – roots are target colour but middle lengths are paler and less golden.
- Solution – apply warmer colour to faded areas.

Basic procedure

1 Apply tint to regrowth. In this case use 9/03 + 30 vol hydrogen peroxide. Develop for 20–25 minutes.
2 Mix fresh tint consisting of 9/04 + 20 vol peroxide. Apply to faded areas. Develop for 5–15 minutes.
3 Shampoo colour from hair and condition.
4 Advise client on home hair-care programme.

8.10 Pre-colouring/pre-pigmentation

Pre-colouring or pre-pigmentation is the technique used to colour pale, porous hair to either darker or redder shades. It is the method of replacing the red pigments which are lost once the hair has been lightened and becomes out of condition.

A typical example of the need to pre-colour hair would be that of a client who has pre-lightened hair and now wishes to return to his or her natural colour. Simply applying a darker tint over the lightened ends would spell disaster! The new colour would look flat (it could even take on a greenish appearance!) and would fade quickly.

Two types of colouring product can be used to pre-colour hair, these being permanent tints and semi-permanent colours.

Choosing the pre-colour

Choose a warm shade 1–3 shades darker than the target colour. The more porous the hair is, the darker and redder the colour should be. Do not choose a colour that contains any ash or mauve.

(a) Using a tint as a pre-colour.
Cream tint – mix 13 cm (5 inches) of colour + 15 ml *water* (no hydrogen peroxide is added).
Liquid tint – mix 2–4 capfuls of colour + 2–4 capfuls *water* (no hydrogen peroxide is added).
(b) Using a semi-permanent product as a pre-colour.
On highly damaged hair, semi-permanent colour molecules will hold in the hair better because they are larger. Semi-permanent colours are also quick and easy to apply.

Perhaps the only disadvantage of using a semi-permanent product as a pre-colour is that you need to be extremely knowledgeable about the range of colours kept in your salon if they do not have a code number. As some semi-permanent colours are described by their name only, they have no code number to tell you the depth and tone of the contents. Only very experienced colourists will usually know, from familiarity with its performance, which semi-permanent product would be the ideal pre-colour to use. For this reason, many hairdressers prefer to use permanent tints for pre-colouring instead.

8.11 Application of pre-colour

Using a tint as a pre-colour

1 Dampen hair and towel-dry thoroughly. (The moisture helps the cuticle to open, ready to absorb the pre-colour.)
2 Apply the pre-colour *sparingly* to the hair to be treated, using either a damp sponge or brush. *Avoid any regrowth*.
3 Work in and distribute the pre-colour through the hair using a fine-toothed comb. (Drying with a hairdrier will help 'lock in' pre-colour.)
4 Apply the target shade directly to the hair over the top of the pre-colour, mixing it with peroxide in the normal way.
5 Allow full development time.

If too much pre-colour is applied, the end result would be either too warm or too dark. Porous hair will absorb the pre-colour quickly. Do not think your application is wrong if the pre-colour gradually fades as you are working; this is just the colour penetrating the hair. The peroxide added to the target shade will activate the pre-colour molecules first, allowing them to lock themselves into the cortex before the target colour molecules.

Using a semi-permanent product as a pre-colour

1 Dampen hair and towel-dry thoroughly.
2 Apply plenty of product to the areas to be pre-coloured, *avoiding any regrowth*.
3 Develop for 10–15 minutes.
4 Rinse and towel-dry thoroughly (or you can leave colour in hair and dry under the drier to help 'lock in' colour).
5 Apply target shade.
6 Allow full development time.

Using a semi-permanent colour is very quick and application is easy. The colour molecules are larger than permanent colour molecules so tend to hold in the hair better. Basic shades are often mixed with warmer colours when using semi-permanent products, to give the pre-colour more depth and tenacity.

N.B. If the previous colour on the hair contains ash, it will be necessary to clean-out this unwanted tone before pre-pigmenting (see [8.4]).

See Case Study (4): Tinting pre-lightened hair darker [8.12].

8.12 Case Study (4): Tinting pre-lightened hair darker

Remember that this example is only a guide and that the application and products you use depend on the hair you are working on and your skill.

- Target colour – 8/3.
- Natural base – dark blonde (base 6/0).
- Condition of hair – porous and damaged.
- Previous colouring – pre-lightener followed by ash toner (depth: 10).
- Problems – hair lacks depth and warmth.
- Solution – clean-out ash toner. Pre-pigment pre-lightened hair.

Basic procedure

1 Do not shampoo or wet hair.
2 Clean-out ash toner from hair using weak mixture of bleach (e.g. powder bleach + 10 vol peroxide). Use cotton wool strips to prevent product from seeping onto regrowth. Develop for 5–10 minutes. Give one gentle shampoo then towel-dry thoroughly.
3 Pre-pigment hair. In this case the following tints were used:

   2 caps of 6/46
   2 caps of 7/44
   plus 4 caps of water

4 Apply tint to regrowth. In this case the following tint was used: 8/3 + 30 vol (9%) hydrogen peroxide. Then the fresh tint mixture was applied immediately to the middle lengths and ends.
5 Apply tint to middle lengths and ends. In this case the following was used: 8/3 + 20 vol hydrogen peroxide.
6 Develop for full development time.
7 Shampoo and condition hair.
8 Advise client on home hair-care programme.

8.13 Subduing unwanted tones in hair (colour neutralization)

In hair colouring, the term 'neutralizing' has nothing to do with what we do to hair when perming. A principle of all colour is that colours opposite each other in the colour circle (Fig. 8.2) will neutralize one another, resulting in a colour with a more subdued tone.

The colour circle consists of three *primary* and three *secondary* colours. The primary colours are red, blue and yellow. They are called primary colours because all other colours can be made when these are mixed. Colours made by mixing the primary colours together are called secondary colours.

Blue and Yellow = Green
Red and Yellow = Orange
Red and Blue = Mauve

In hair colouring, hairdressers must be familiar with the colour circle so that the correct colour is chosen for subduing any unwanted tones.

Colours opposite each other in the colour circle will neutralize each other thus:

Orange will be neutralized by blue
Yellow will be neutralized by mauve
Orange-yellow will be neutralized by bluish-mauve

Perhaps it is now easy for you to understand why hair turns green! A hairdresser (or client!) may use a blue-based ash on very yellow hair thinking it will eliminate the yellow. Instead they end up with hair which is green! (Blue + yellow = green.) What should be used instead?

Mix primary colours to obtain secondary colours.

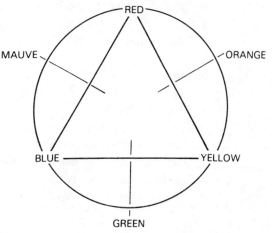

Fig. 8.2 The colour circle.

You must become familiar with the manufacturers' numbering systems for colouring products used in your salon, so that you can identify what colours are contained in them. Without this knowledge, you will be unable to select the correct colour needed to neutralize unwanted tones in hair.

See Case Study (5): Examples of controlling unwanted tones in hair [8.14].

8.14 Case Study (5): Examples of controlling unwanted tones in hair

Remember that these examples should be regarded as a guide only and that the application and products you use depend upon the hair you are working on and your skill.

Example 1:

- Target colour – basic shade to cover white hair.
- Natural base – light warm brown.
- Problem – basic shade turns out golden.
- Solution – use corresponding shade containing ash.
- Result – basic shade.

Example 2:

- Target colour – basic light blonde.
- Natural base – dark blonde.
- Problem – lengths and ends yellow from sun.
- Solution – use a mauve ash to neutralize yellow.
- Result – basic light blonde.

Example 3:

- Target – silver.
- Natural base – 100% white.
- Problem – pollution, etc. has caused the hair to yellow. (Smoke from cigarettes may cause the front hair-line to yellow.)
- Solution – use a silver temporary colour.
- Result – excess yellow will be neutralized.

8.15 Lightening already pre-lightened hair

Sometimes clients who have had their hair pre-lightened to a yellow base will ask if they can go even lighter, to a vary pale creamy blonde.

Doing this is not as simple as running the bleach through the lengths and ends for the last 10–15 minutes of development time. Yellow pigment is diffuse. This means that the molecules of pigment are small and therefore difficult to remove. We have all experienced the bleach highlights that seem to take forever to lighten from yellow to very pale yellow. Figure 8.3 shows how long the development takes:

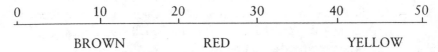

Fig. 8.3 Approximately how long development takes during pre-lightening (in minutes).

Because yellow pigment is diffuse and therefore stubborn and hard to eliminate, a *stronger* bleaching mixture is required. But the hair must be in good enough condition to take this treatment. If you think the hair is not in a good enough state, renegotiate the target colour with the client.

See Case Study (6): Lightening already pre-lightened hair [8.16].

8.16 Case Study (6): Lightening already pre-lightened hair

Remember that this example should be regarded as a guide only and that the application and products you use depend on the hair you are working on and your skill.

- Target colour – very pale ash blonde.
- Natural base – light brown.
- Condition of hair – able to take further pre-lightening.
- Previous colouring – pre-lightener (to yellow base) followed by golden blonde toner.
- Problems – hair unable to take target colour without further pre-lightening.
- Solution – lighten lengths and ends further using pre-lightener.

Adjust strength of product and development time for regrowth according to colour requirements.

Basic procedure

1 Apply appropriate strength pre-lightener to regrowth. Start development time.
2 Mix a pre-lightener *stronger* than the one you have used on the regrowth. (Powder bleach is ideal for this.)
3 Apply stronger pre-lightener to the lengths and ends about half-way through the roots' development time.
4 Keep an eye on the lengths and ends – they may lighten suddenly. If this happens, the pre-lightener may need to be removed before the roots have completed their development. (If this is the case, use a bowl of water and cotton wool to remove the pre-lightener from the lengths and ends, without disturbing product on regrowth.)
5 Rinse and shampoo gently.
6 Apply toner in normal way. Develop toner.
7 Rinse, shampoo and condition hair.
8 Advise client on home hair-care programme.

8.17 Correcting highlights and lowlights

There are two main ways of highlighting or lowlighting hair:

(1) The weave method (foil and Easi-Meche);
(2) The cap or plastic bag method.

Mistakes can, and do, happen, and you need to know how to put them right, whether it is your mistake, the client's, or another hairdresser's. Figure 8.4 sets out suitable ways of dealing with these problems.

Corrective colouring can be very time-consuming. If, for example, patches of bleach are caused by leakage or seepage, you may need to pre-pigment those areas before applying a colour to reproduce the client's natural shade. However, if just a natural shade is applied to the patches, it will disguise the mistake but will probably fade quickly.

8.18 Hair after-care routines

Clients seem to learn more about personal hair-care from magazines and television commercials than they do from their

Problem	Possible causes	Solution
Colour does not show	Either: (a) Bright enough colour was not achieved; or (b) Too few strands were coloured.	Repeat colouring procedure. If you are using a pre-lightener, avoid using on the already pre-lightened hair where possible.
Too many highlights or lowlights	Either: (a) Too strong a colour was achieved giving the illusion of more highlights or lowlights; or (b) Too much hair was coloured.	Select strands by weave method and apply a tint which will reproduce the cllient's natural shade. This will disguise some of the coloured hair, making the natural shade show more.
Wrong tone	Either: (a) Wrong choice of colour used; or (b) Product was not allowed to develop to intended shade.	Either: (a) Correct by using a semi-permanent; or (b) Apply toner over entire hair. (If it is an oxidation toner, do not allow to stay on long enough to affect natural shade.)
Patches of colour at roots	Either: (a) Foil packages have leaked; or (b) Product has seeped through cap or plastic bag.	Go through hair and apply a colour to reproduce the client's natural shade. (N.B. As the tint will be in contact with the skin, ensure a skin test has been carried out previous to this application, if necessary.)

Fig. 8.4 Correcting highlights and lowlights – at a glance.

hairdressers! Educate your clients about their hair, give them tips on its styling for use between salon visits and recommend the hair products they need to maintain its style and condition. If possible, display these products in the salon so that the client can buy what you recommend from the salon instead of the chemist's shop. This practice will increase the salon's profits, encourage your client to value your judgement and also help your client's hair look better between visits to the salon. What could be a better advertisement for you and your salon than people complimenting your client about her hair and then asking for the salon's telephone number?

- Recommend cleansing, conditioning and styling products and explain what benefits they will have.
- Suggest that styling methods should not include the use of excessive heat and harsh treatment (for example, very hot tongs or the regular and frequent use of heated rollers), to prevent further physical damage to the hair.
- Explain that hair should be thoroughly rinsed with water after

swimming in the sea or swimming pools treated with chlorine, as both of these make hair dry.

- Explain that the sun's rays will bleach hair and make it dry when sun-bathing. Suggest that something should be worn to protect the hair such as a hat or scarf, or that a product specifically designed as a sun-blocker for the hair should be applied.

8.19   Revision questions

1   What are the three changes that can be made to hair colour?
2   What is the most limiting factor to be considered when corrective colouring is necessary?
3   What technique is used to remove mild colour build-up from the lengths and ends of hair, or toners from bleached hair?
4   Why is the result of a colour stripper often uneven?
5   When is pre-pigmentation necessary?
6   What types of colorants can be used for pre-pigmentation?
7   In the colour circle, what is the opposite colour to:

(a)   blue?
(b)   green?
(c)   yellow?

8   A client returns to the salon to complain that her highlights do not show. What could be the possible reasons for this?
9   What determines the choice of colour to be used for pre-pigmentation?
10   How is a tint applied when it is being used for pre-pigmenting the hair?

8.20 Advanced questions

1   Describe the procedure (step by step) for removing an unwanted dark tint from hair.
2   Explain why pre-pigmenting is necessary when tinting bleached hair back to its natural colour.
3   Describe how you would correct a set of weave highlights which had resulted in unsightly patches of lightened hair at the roots.
4   Describe how you would even out the colour of the lengths and ends of tinted hair which showed:

(a)   minimal fade
(b)   excessive fade.

9

Creative Colouring
Techniques

9.1 Selective/partial colouring techniques

Partial colouring, or using different colours in the hair, can be used to enhance specific areas of a haircut and to add texture to the finished style. This type of colouring has become increasingly popular for the following reasons:

- Most techniques will not give a regrowth and some are even removed with the next haircut.
- It can be subtle or bold.
- Partial colouring introduces shy clients to using colour.
- It stimulates interest amongst staff and clients.
- It provides a personalized colour technique for the client.
- It is inexpensive when compared to whole head colouring.

Clients are attracted to unusual happenings, so you can afford to show off a little – the attention will help increase turnover.

Basically it is only your imagination that limits how you choose to apply colour to hair. Inspiration will come from looking at things around you. Just because it hasn't been done before doesn't mean it isn't possible – so experiment! Look at the feathers on a bird, the fur on an animal, how leaves have dark and light patterns. Visit art galleries and look closely at paintings to see how the artist uses colour to create shadows, highlights and texture.

The last thing you should do is believe that because a client has booked only for a cut and blow dry, he or she is not willing to have a colour treatment. Most can be easily persuaded to have subtle colouring if it does not involve long-term commitment.

Block colouring and touch colouring are examples of techniques that you could try.

9.2 Block colouring

What is it?

Block colouring is when specific areas of a haircut are emphasized by the use of colour. This technique lends itself very well to styles such as the 'Wedge' and 'Firefly' because the short sides on both of these haircuts can be darkened to add interest to these areas. Alternatively, this technique can be used to soften the hard straight lines of a bob (Fig. 9.1).

How is it done?

The hair must already be cut and styled. Choose colours that will complement the hair you will *not* be colouring. Section areas using zig-zag partings to avoid hard lines in the final result. Apply your colorant and allow to process. For block colouring a bob, take a fine mesh above the chosen area to be coloured. This will avoid any harsh lines in the final result as the fine mesh will lie over the coloured hair.

9.3 Touch colouring

What is it?

Touch colouring is a technique that creates the same effect as the sun, lightening the ends of the hair. Powder bleach is used to achieve this.

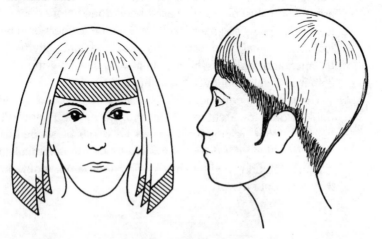

Fig. 9.1 Block colouring.

How is it done?

Liberally apply hairspray to the roots of the hair to hold it away from the scalp. Longer hair may need backcombing before spraying. Apply the pre-lightener with the fingers to the tips of the hair.

9.4 Imaginative application techniques

You can use almost *anything* to put colour onto hair. Here are a few ideas, but they are by no means the only methods.

Combs

By using different combs that have a variation of space between the teeth, you can comb colour onto the hair in varying amounts. Either dip the comb into the colorant or put the colorant onto the comb with a tint brush. Place the colour exactly where you want it, emphasizing specific areas of the haircut.

Brushes

The most suitable brushes are the open type (e.g. vent brush) as they have rounded 'bristles'.

Dip the brush into the colorant and then gently 'pat' the hair with the brush. If you use several shades you can achieve a marvellous tortoise-shell effect. This is a fairly subtle way of getting colour onto the hair – so don't be too cautious about the colour choice.

You can also use paint-brushes and toothbrushes (clean, of course!). These give variation in the amount of colour applied.

Fingers

Dip your gloved fingers into the tint or bleach and then 'paint' the hair. Another way is to put a brushful of colorant into the gloved palm of the hand and gently squeeze your hand to make a fist (this distributes the colour), then 'scrunch' the colour onto the hair. This gives a delightful 'cobweb' effect, particularly if using bleach.

Hair clamps and clips

Dip the hair clamp into the colorant and then attach it to the hair at an appropriate point – you can use several clamps. Leave the clamp in position during the development of the colour. This is a very effective way of creating flecks of colour in the hair.

Applicator bottles, icing bags or syringes

Fill the applicator or icing bag with the colorant (gel-based products are best, since the cream types are too thick). You then 'pipe' a pattern onto the hair. This gives a speckled effect – or you can achieve specific patterns if you use this technique with stronger colours.

Water sprays and airbrushes

An airbrush is a special drawing instrument used by artists. It sprays colour onto a surface and it can be adapted for use with hair colour. Colorant is put into a pressurized container and is then forced through a fine nozzle. This enables you to spray colour onto a particular part of the haircut.

Water sprays can also be adapted for this technique – but check that the nozzle is fine enough. This is a particularly effective technique when used on very light hair. You can achieve fantastic 'mother of pearl' effects if you use several colours (diluted food colours work especially well) and merge one colour into another. High volume strength hydrogen peroxide used in a water spray and then lightly sprayed over dark hair will give a very delicate bronzed effect – *but be careful* – you must protect the client's skin and clothing and make sure you remove the hydrogen peroxide from the water spray when finished!

Stencils

Cut out the desired shape, using thin flexible sheets of plastic or cardboard. Secure this firmly to the hair in the appropriate position using clips. Apply plenty of product to the unmasked shape and leave to process. This is a very effective method of achieving specific shapes or patterns on the hair. It works best on straight hair.

Foil and Easi-Meche

Besides conventional highlighting techniques you can use foil in other ways. Tear a strip of foil (about 10 × 25 cm). Apply the colorant heavily onto the foil. Hold the foil at each end and then wipe across the hair.

If using two or three colours, use a 'shoe-shine' movement across the hair. You will achieve a lovely tortoise-shell, mottled effect. This works best on shorter hair.

Another method is to place a mesh of hair onto the foil. Put two or three colours onto the hair, overlapping one onto the other. Enclose the mesh in the foil to develop. This gives a strong mottled effect.

Corrugated cardboard

Use small pieces of cardboard (approximately $10 \times 15\,\text{cm}$). Apply several colours along the grooves of the cardboard. Place a mesh of hair onto the cardboard and then cover it with another piece. Secure the two pieces firmly together, using clothes pegs or hair clips. This works best on longer hair, giving a dappled effect.

Framing

This is a way of applying colour to the hair to produce uniform lines of colour. Simply take a circular frame of approximately 40 cm in diameter and thread through pieces of natural fibre string (how many you use and the thickness of the string should be developed by experimentation). Apply the colorant generously to the string using a brush. It can be applied to the hair in a number of ways – so experiment. You can simply press the string against the hair to leave short lines of colour, or you can press the left sides of string against the hair and gradually 'roll' the frame until the strings on the right side are in contact with the hair. You can achieve a band of colour around the hair by careful positioning of the frame.

9.5   Promoting hair colour in the salon

Colour can be a profitable part of your business. Clients who are satisfied with colour results tend to be loyal to the salon for a long time.

To promote the use of colour in your salon, keep the following points in mind:

- *Talk about colour* with your clients. Generally speaking, we have the client's undivided attention for at least half an hour – so use this time constructively to create more colour business.

- *Visuals such as fashionable pictures* around the salon are often more useful than colour charts because clients relate more to these.
- *Staff should wear colour* in their hair. Nothing advertises the use of colour better than seeing it 'in the flesh'.
- *Display colouring products* that the client can buy from the salon for home use. These might include colour sprays, gels and mousses.
- *Consultations take time so allow for plenty of discussion* with the client, using visuals such as charts, pictures and staff's hair.
- *Show off a little* when using colour in an interesting way in the salon. People are inquisitive and they will ask what is happening to the client next to them.
- *Learn all you can about hair colour* and the newest techniques. If you do not know about it you cannot talk confidently to your clients.

9.6   Selling hair colour in the salon

Hairdressers often miss golden opportunities to sell hair colour to clients. Why does this happen? Perhaps the best way of analysing this situation is to understand a little of the psychology of selling. Imagine that a client has booked an appointment for a cut and blow dry. While you are looking at his or her hair and discussing the style, your judgement tells you that the hair would look even better if it was given a set of foil highlights. You suggest this and the possible responses of the client are shown in Fig. 9.2.

As you can see from the diagram, most clients fall into the 'lukewarm' category, and it is your influence on such clients that can sell the service. You should never push a client into having a service they neither want, need nor can afford – this is bad selling and is ultimately bad for business. Clients should always feel at ease or they will not return. If the service you are selling will be of benefit to the client's appearance and hair, your interest will be appreciated.

The process of selling can be divided into three steps:

(1)   Analysing the client's needs;
(2)   Giving advice (introducing the service);
(3)   Gaining agreement on how to meet these needs.

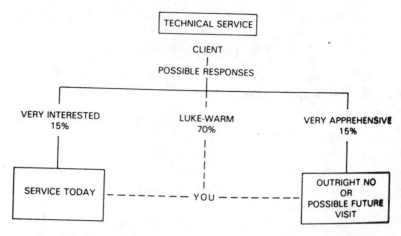

Fig. 9.2 The possible responses of a client to extra services. (Courtesy L'Oréal.)

Let's look at these steps in more detail.

Analysing the client's needs

- Establish a relationship by developing interest and trust;
- Ask open questions which begin with How? When? Where? Why? and Which?;
- Demonstrate understanding by using visual aids such as shade charts;
- Formulate an opinion based on sound technical knowledge of colouring services.

Giving advice

- Explain the service in terms of what it will do for the client;
- Convince the client of these benefits;
- Be enthusiastic and have a positive belief in what you are recommending.

Gaining agreement

- Suggest the service is given at that moment;
- Reassure the client if still apprehensive and perhaps suggest alternatives.

People say that they have 'seen it all before' – show them that
they haven't!
Enjoy your work – colouring is fun!

9.7 Revision questions

1 List six reasons why partial colouring techniques are popular
   with clients.
2 When using the block colouring technique, why are zig-zag
   partings used to divide the hair?
3 List four creative colouring techniques and explain how each
   one is carried out.
4 How can hair colouring be promoted in the salon?

9.8 Advanced questions

1 Explain how you would train new and junior staff to promote
   hair colouring services in the salon.
2 Describe how you would plan a two-week colour promotion in
   order to increase salon turnover.
3 Select two creative colouring techniques and write step-by-step
   explanatory notes to be used as training material for new and
   junior staff.
4 Devise a 'benefits' list for each creative colouring technique
   that could be used as part of a training session for staff.

A Brief History of Hair Colouring

10.1 Ancient civilisations

The use of henna for colouring hair goes back thousands of years. Henna powders have been found in the ancient tombs of Pharoahs in Egypt alongside perfumes and make-up products of that age. As long ago as 2000 BC, Egyptians mixed henna powder (obtained by grinding the leaves of the *Lawsonia inermis* bush shown in Fig. 10.1) with other vegetable extracts and metallic compounds to change their hair colour.

The ingredients would be mixed to a smooth paste using very hot water and perfumed oils, before being applied to the hair. The client sat in the hot sun until the henna paste dried to form a hard crust. The dried henna paste was then rinsed from the hair.

The addition of such substances as animal blood and indigo deepened the red hue of the henna and was popular with Egyptian men for darkening their greying beards. It is believed that one Egyptian dignitary had the blood of a black cow boiled with henna powder and oils in the belief that the blood from a black cow would be darker and help restore a more natural colour to his greying beard!

Hair colouring preparations made from white lead and vermillion have also been found in Greek tombs. This concoction would deepen the hair colour and add redness.

Virtually every Roman writer mentioned the fashionable use of hair colour. Torok wrote 'they blackened their eyebrows with soot or charred ant eggs; to dye their hair, they used a walnut strain and lead or copper acetate'. Dark hair was fashionable in ancient Rome until Caesar returned with his entourage of blonde-haired females captured from Gaul (ancient France). Their blonde hair was a revelation to the dark-haired women of Rome. The blonde captives were scorned for their new source of physical attraction and were called *pictae* (painted women). The aristocratic women had wigs made from the hair of the pictae and also applied a variety of pastes and lotions made from elderberries, nutshells and

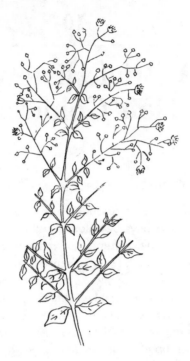

Fig. 10.1   Lawsonia inermis.

vinegar sediment to their hair in order to lighten it. Martial, a writer of that time, wrote the following verse:

'The golden hair that Galla wears
Is hers – who would have thought it?
She swears 'tis hers, and true she swears
For I know where she bought it.'

10.2 The Renaissance

Blonde hair became fashionable again in Italy during the Renaissance period. To lighten their naturally dark hair, elegant Venetian women would sit in the sun, wearing a hat with no crown, with their hair spread over the wide brim. This is shown in Fig. 10.2. The hat, called a *solana* served as a baking platform for the hair which was coated with mixtures of alum, black sulphur and honey, and as a parasol to shield their bodies from the sun.

Special sun terraces were built on the tops of houses where women would practise *arte biondegiante* which would preoccupy them for three or four hours during the hottest part of the day. The

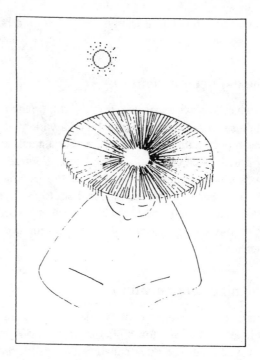

Fig. 10.2 Arte biondegiante – wearing a solana.

Venetian blonde colouring, achieved by the arte biondegiante method was immortalized by the artists Titian and Tintoretto, and was introduced to France by Marguerite de Valois, a woman renowned for constantly changing her hair colour.

10.3 The seventeenth century

During the seventeenth century, many English women dyed their hair red in honour of Elizabeth I. They achieved this by soaking their hair in a solution of alum followed by a rinse made from rhubarb. In 1694, *The Ladies Dictionary* was published in London claiming to be 'A Work Never Attempted before in English'. Under the heading *Hair, grey or otherwise, to make it black* was written:

'Hair to render it black, take the Bark of Oak Root, the Green Husks of Walnuts, three ounces of each, the deepest and oldest Red-Wine a Port, boil them, bruised and well mixed to the Consumption of half a Pint, strain out the juice, and adde of the Oyl of Myrtle a pound and a half, set them for six days in the Sun in a Leaden Mortar, stirring them well, add the annointing the Hair, it will turn any Coloured hair as black as Jet in often doing.'

10.4 The eighteenth century

The wearing of wigs was very popular during the eighteenth century and these were powdered to achieve a variety of colours. In 1789, it was reported that 24 million pounds of starch were used to make hair powder every year. In 1795, England introduced a tax on hair powders which required wearers of the powder to purchase an annual certificate. This certificate had to be shown to the hairdresser before hair powder was applied. Needless to say, the fashion of wearing hair powder was soon replaced by more natural hairstyles!

10.5 The nineteenth century

During the nineteenth century, dark brown and black hair were fashionable. In *The Art of Perfumary*, G.W. Septimus informed readers of a new hair dye called *Baffine* produced by Mr Condy of Battersea. Mr Septimus wrote:

> 'Baffine . . . is a solution of permanganate of potash. This salt, like nitrate of silver, undergoes a decomposition when in contact with organic substances. Hair and skin are stained by it of a good chestnut hue.'

Hydrogen peroxide was discovered in 1818 and was first used to lighten hair in 1860 by Cora Pearl, mistress of Napoleon II. At the International Exhibition held in Paris in 1867, the use of hydrogen peroxide to lighten hair was demonstrated by London chemist E.H. Thiellay and Parisian hairdresser Léon Hugot. They called their lotion *Eau de fontaine de Jouvence dorée* (Golden water from the fountain of youth). It was in fact nothing more than a 3% (10 vol) hydrogen peroxide solution.

In 1863, Haussman, a man employed in the dyeing of animal fibres, discovered paraphenylenediamine, one of the first synthetic dyes. It was not until 1883, that Haussman discovered this new dye substance could be used for the colouring of human hair too. There was nothing to stop the natural progression and development of synthetic hair colorants from this point onwards.

10.6   The twentieth century

Up until the 1920s, synthetic oxidation dyes were used mainly to conceal white hair but this era brought a new sense of freedom for women and new fashions in hair. Oxidation dyes were greatly improved and the barriers of convention broken down to create a boom in hair colouring.

During the 1940s, the use of bleach and temporary colours were all the rage, influenced by Hollywood stars such as Lana Turner. By the end of World War II (1945), a lot of new colorants had been developed (including those for home use) providing a wide colour choice. In 1951, *Life Magazine* reported 'since the development of home hair dyes, about one woman in five has taken to some kind of touching up'.

By the 1960s, the use of hair colorants was very popular and the American *Cosmopolitan* magazine stated 'The day of the mousy blonde has passed, as has the era of the platinum blonde, the carrot redhead, the shoe-polish brunette'. *Cosmopolitan* went on to say that 'the modern woman's hair had turned Just Peachy, Copper Blaze, White Minx, Chocolate Kiss, Fushia, Honey Doux, Bordeaux, Fury and Frivolous Fawn'. New colouring techniques were also launched in the 1960s. *Drabbing* was used for toning down bright colours (especially reds and yellows) by application of white or champagne-coloured rinses. *Frosting* involved bleaching small strands of top hair all over the head while *tipping* was bleaching the strands of hair that framed the face. The technique of *streaking* was the bleaching of several broad streaks of hair starting at the front hairline around the face.

The 1970's colourist used stencils to add colour to hairstyles which were worn straight or flat. Another popular technique was adding large areas of different colours to fringes, or colouring wide stripes on either side of a parting. The *punk* revolution which happened during the late 1970s also meant the popular use of strong pink, red, orange and yellow hair colour. These bold colouring techniques were replaced in the 1980s by much more subtle techniques. These included *naturalizing* and *tortoiseshell* highlights which result in several complementary shades and tones being put in the hair by weaving out selected strands for colouring.

10.7   Hair colouring today

It was not so long ago, that there was considerable public prejudice against women (let alone men) using any form of hair colorant. At best, tinting was used for disguising white hair, using black or brown dyes. However, with the increasing readiness of society to accept hair colouring as part of the total grooming process for both men and women, more hair colouring is undertaken today than ever before. Clients no longer look upon their hair colour as 'something to be made the best of', but as a definite asset that can improve their overall appearance and, in some cases, their social and career success. In fact, hair colour can make such a statement that it is often used by performers and celebrities to attract attention and to create a trademark.

The development of hair colouring products and new application techniques in recent times has been truly phenomenal. As a result, many hairdressers now specialize as hair colour technicians. Hairdressers owe a great deal to the chemists who develop the excellent colouring products with which we work today and to the hair colour experts of the industry who so willingly share their ideas and pass on their skills.

Glossary

accelerator: infra-red heater to speed up processing time.

acid-balanced: pH same as hair and skin (4.5–5.5).

aftercare: maintenance of hairstyle and condition between visits to the salon.

albino: a person whose hair and skin lack pigment.

ammonium carbonate: active part of powder bleach which speeds release of oxygen.

ammonium hydroxide: (ammonia) alkaline chemical in tint and bleaching, used as a catalyst.

analysis: pre-examination of the scalp and hair before colouring/processing.

aniline dyes: colorants made from coal derivatives.

anthraquinones: dyes contained in some semi-permanents.

anti-oxidant: acid rinse which reduces subsequent oxidation damage. Ascorbic acid is an example of an anti-oxidant.

application: putting colorant on all or part of the hair.

ash: shades containing blue or violet; opposite to 'warm'.

azo-dyes: dyes contained in some temporary colours.

basic shade: manufacturer's shade of tint which contains either no tone or very little.

band: overlap onto previously tinted hair will cause this when tinting a regrowth.

beige: neither ash nor gold; a mixture of both tones.

bleach: product capable of lightening the hair.

blonde: light hair colour.

booster: chemicals (persulphates) which give extra oxygen in bleaching.

calamine lotion: a lotion which can help soothe irritated and sore skin. It can be applied to a skin test area following a positive reaction.

camomile: vegetable colorant, mainly used on blonde hair.

canities: hair that grows without colour; white hair.

cap highlights: method of highlighting using a special rubber cap.

catalyst: agent which speeds up a chemical reaction while itself remaining unchanged in the process.

cendré: containing blue or violet; opposite to 'warm'. (French for ash.)

cleaning-out: removing unwanted colour by applying a bleach.

colour circle: shows primary and secondary colours. Used for the selection of correct colours when subduing unwanted tones in hair.

colour reducers: products that strip unwanted artificial colour from hair.

compatible: able to mix without a violent reaction.

compound colorant: mixture of vegetable and mineral. Compound henna is a mixture of henna and a metallic salt.

concentrate: strong colour solution which can be diluted.

contra-indication: indication against performing colouring.

controller: same as booster.

cool colour: same as cendré.

corrective colouring: rectifying unwanted results.

cortex: middle layer of hair. Consists of bundles of fibres and contains natural hair colour. The cortex is the part of the hair where chemical changes take place.

cosmetic colorant: (quasi-permanent) type of colorant which is a cross between a semi-permanent and permanent oxidation colorant.

crayon: form of temporary colour.

cream tint: type of colour usually packaged in tubes.

cuticle: outside layer of hair which protects the cortex beneath it. Consists of several layers.

depth: how light or how dark the hair is. This is described on a scale of 1–10 or 2–11.

dermal papilla: collection of cells at the base of the follicle which is the source of hair growth.

dermatitis: inflammation of the skin as a result of being in contact with some external agent, such as para-based colorants.

dermis: internal layer of skin, lying below the epidermis and containing blood vessels and nerve endings. Hair follicles and glands are found here.

develop: process of colour forming.

development time: time (recommended by the product manufacturers) that a colorant is left on the hair to enable the colour to form.

drab: matt, dull, ash, flat.

Easi-Meche: self-sealing plastic packets used for fashion colouring. Manufactured by L'Oréal.

elasticity test: tests cortex for internal damage by stretching the hair between the fingers. Hair in good condition will stretch 30% of its length.

emulsify: in colouring, process of loosening colour from hair and scalp by massage.

emulsion bleach: type of pre-lightener.

epidermis: outer layer of skin. Hair follicles and sweat glands are downgrowths of the epidermis. Contains no blood vessels or nerves.

fade: when the intensity of a colour diminishes.

fastness: how well a colour resists fade.

fluorescent lighting: strip lighting; some tubes (warm white) give out light which is approximately equal to daylight.

foil: thin sheet of aluminium which is used for weave highlights.

follicle: minute pit in epidermis from which hair grows.

frosting: strands of lightened hair.

grab: when a colour is held by hair longer than expected. If, for instance, a temporary colour is 'grabbed' it will last longer than one shampoo.

grey hair: a mixture of white and coloured hairs.

hair: form of keratin which grows from the follicle.

hair growth cycle: describes the three stages of the growth of a hair.

henna: vegetable colour which gives a regrowth. Derived from *Lawsonia inermis*.

highlighting: lightening selected strands of hair.

hydrogen peroxide: chemical source of oxygen for tinting and lightening processes.

ICC: International Colour Code system.

incompatibility test: test to determine whether damage would be caused by using a product system containing hydrogen peroxide. Metallic salts would cause a violent chemical reaction with hydrogen peroxide.

incompatible: a chemical reaction causing damage to the hair/ scalp.

infra-red: invisible form of radiation which gives off heat. Used to accelerate the development of tints.

intensity: degree of colour brightness.

keratin: protein which forms hair, skin and nails. Different from other proteins in that it contains sulphur.

keratinization: process of keratin formation.

lawsone: the active ingredient of henna.

lawsonia inermis: plant which is source of henna. Leaves are ground into a fine powder to give lawsone.

lightening: removal of colour.

lightening setting lotion: setting lotion containing hydrogen peroxide.

lightening shampoo: a weak oxidant mixture which lightens hair.

lightening tint: tint capable of lifting up to four shades on the depth scale. Usually suitable only on hair which has a natural depth of six or lighter.

lowlighting: darkening of selected strands of hair.

matt: drab, dull, flat. Light rays are scattered instead of reflected so the hair will not shine.

medulla: centre of hair, consisting of hollow air spaces. Not present in all hair.

melanin: black and brown pigment found in cortex of hair and also the skin.

melanocytes: cells in the hair and epidermis which produce melanin.

metallic colorants: hair colorants containing metallic salts.

mitosis: type of cell division where one cell divides to give two copies of itself.

ml: millilitre; metric unit for measuring volume (one-thousandth of a litre); same as cc (cubic centimetre).

molecule: smallest particle of a colorant that can exist on its own.

mordant: chemical used with or added to colours to fix them to hair.

mousse: foam-based product available in coloured forms.

neutralize: term used for cancelling of unwanted colours.

nitro-dyes: chemicals used in semi-permanent colours.

oil bleach: mild bleach product with added oils which is capable of up to four shades of lift.

opaque: allows no light to pass through.

opposite colours: colours which neutralize each other (*see* colour circle).

overlapping: when doing a regrowth, colorant is incorrectly applied onto previously coloured hair, causing bands of darker hair when tinting, and possible breakage when bleaching.

overprocessed: overdevelopment of chemical products, resulting in poor results or damage.

oxidants/oxidizers: chemicals which add oxygen thereby causing a change in the colour molecules when tinting and bleaching.

oxidation: chemical process by which oxygen is added (or hydrogen is removed).

paints: form of temporary colour which is applied to dry hair after styling.

papilla: source of hair growth found at the base of the follicle.

para-compounds: chemicals used in permanent/quasi colours (also in some semi-permanents) – paraphenylenediamine and paratoluenediamine. Mixed with hydrogen peroxide to develop colour in cortex of hair.

patch test: another name for skin test.

permanent colour: colorant which gives a regrowth (tint and henna). The colour is not removed by shampooing.

peroxometer: instrument used to measure volume or percentage strength of hydrogen peroxide. Measures the relative density of the peroxide.

persulphates: chemicals which give off oxygen. Used as boosters to give extra oxygen in bleaching.

pH: (potential of hydrogen) symbol for hydrogen concentration; a scale of numbers tells you exactly how acid or alkaline something is.

pheomelanin: red and yellow pigment of hair, found in cortex.

porosity test: test to assess condition of cuticle.

porous: hair with an open cuticle, able to absorb liquids.

powder bleach: form of bleach mixed with hydrogen peroxide to form a paste (also known as paste bleach).

pre-disposition test: another name for skin test (American).

pre-lightening: alternative name for bleaching.

pre-pigmentation: replacement of lost pigment caused by lightening or colour fade.

pre-softening: applying hydrogen peroxide to hair to lift cuticle scales.

primary colours: colours from which all other colours can be made, namely red, blue and yellow.

processing: chemical reaction in hair which brings about a permanent change, such as bleaching or tinting.

progressive: gradual development of colour; does not give immediate result.

quaternary ammonium compounds: type of detergent with positive charge; can be used as shampoo or conditioner. Cetrimide is an example which is found in shampoos, conditioners and antiseptics.

quasi-permanent colorant: term for colour product in between semi-permanent and permanent because the colour will gradually fade each time the hair is shampooed, but it also gives a regrowth.

receptive: hair which accepts colour readily.

record card: means of recording clients' colour treatments.

reducer: product used to remove artificial colour from hair.

reduction: process of adding hydrogen or taking away oxygen.

regrowth: new hair growth after tinting or bleaching.

resistant: hair which does not accept colour easily.

rinse: type of temporary colour.

Sabourand-Rousseau test: same as skin test; named after the inventor of the test.

sebaceous gland: gland which produces sebum; attached to the side of the follicle.

sebum: naturally occurring oil of skin and hair, produced by the sebaceous gland.

secondary colours: colours which are made from mixing two primary colours together.

semi-permanent: colour which gradually fades; lasts 4–6 shampoos.

sensitivity test: same as skin test.

shade: depth, tone and intensity of colour.

shade chart: manufacturer's guide to available colours.

skin test: test to show whether a client's skin would react to a colorant containing para-compounds and carried out before application of certain colorants.

spatula: implement with flat surface, used to lay strands of hair on for colour application.

spectrum: seven colours from which white light is made. Seen in the rainbow.

stabilizer: chemicals used to stop a product from deteriorating.

strand test: test to check and monitor colour results.

streaking: alternative name for highlighting.

stripping: removal of unwanted artificial colour.

synthetic: artificial colorant.

target colour: the colour you are aiming for.

temporary colour: colour which lasts until the hair is next shampooed.

test cutting: (or colour test) test to determine if proposed coloration should be performed. It is carried out on a small sample cutting of the client's hair.

tint: permanent colour.

tone: the colour (and its intensity) we see in hair, e.g. copper, gold, ash, red, etc. The character of the colour.

toner: colorant used to add tone after bleaching. This can be a temporary, semi/quasi permanent or permanent colour.

translucent: allows some light to pass through.

transparent: allows all light to pass through. Opposite to opaque.

tungsten filament lighting: somewhat yellowish light given out by light bulbs which have a tungsten filament. The filament heats up to become incandescent and give out light.

ultra-violet rays: invisible form of radiation which causes melanin to be produced in the skin. Can burn the skin and damage the eyes.

underdeveloped: insufficient processing of colour.

uneven colour: colour result is not uniform; varies along hair length or in specific areas.

vegetable colorants: natural colour products derived from plants such as henna and camomile.

vibrance: brightness and intensity of colour.

virgin hair: hair which has not been previously chemically processed.

warm colours: red, gold, yellow or copper.

weave colouring: technique used to select strands of hair for colouring, i.e. highlights or lowlights.

white hair: hair which contains no pigment.

white light: the result of mixing the seven spectral colours (red, orange, yellow, green, blue, indigo, violet).

Index